Using Medicines Information

No. 9 in the Harnessing Health Information series

Series Editor

MICHAEL RIGBY

Using Medicines Information

Edited by

CHRISTINE BOND

Professor of Primary Care (Pharmacy)
University of Aberdeen

Foreword by

ANN LEWIS

Secretary and Registrar
Royal Pharmaceutical Society of Great Britain

Radcliffe Publishing
Oxford • New York

Radcliffe Publishing Ltd
18 Marcham Road
Abingdon
Oxon OX14 1AA
United Kingdom

www.radcliffe-oxford.com

Electronic catalogue and worldwide online ordering facility.

British Library Cataloguing in Publication Data

A catalogue record for this book is available from the British Library.

ISBN-13: 978 1 85775 690 6

Typeset by Pindar New Zealand (Egan Reid), Auckland, New Zealand
Printed and bound by TJI Digital, Padstow, Cornwall, UK

Contents

Foreword

This book resulted from a chance meeting with Michael Rigby the Editor of the series with whom I had worked some years previously. When he told me about his work on the series we discussed the possibility of including a book on medicines information to fill a current gap. I agreed to find an editor. I was delighted when Christine Bond agreed to take on the task. Christine is an established author and editor and we all share an interest in optimising the use of information for the benefit of healthcare so this was a happy alliance. Everyone uses information – not only healthcare professionals and managers but also patients and the public. For all of these people information should be easy to assimilate and to understand.

New technologies have had as significant an impact on methods of communication as on treatment. The development of electronic means of communication, data storage and retrieval has increased the availability of information, requiring new approaches to managing and using it. Similarly new technologies have led to the development of new and complex medicines opening up new opportunities for treatment which require information and explanation.

Medicines are the most common therapeutic intervention in healthcare. This book *Using Medicines Information* is both necessary and timely. Christine Bond has drawn together a number of expert contributors on a carefully selected series of topics which take the reader from availability and supply through considerations for rational and cost effective use to monitoring for both outcome and safety.

In the present policy climate which recognises the need for choice and access, this volume can be recommended to those with an interest in medicines and their use. Serendipity has resulted in many good things, this book fulfils a need and will, I hope, be the first of many editions.

Ann Lewis
Secretary and Registrar
Royal Pharmaceutical Society of Great Britain
August 2007

Preface

I am delighted to have been asked to edit this book on *Using Medicines Information* as part of the *Harnessing Health Information Series*. So much of health now depends on the use of medicines, either to prevent future health-related events, or to treat existing conditions. There is also a general interest in lifestyle drugs and options for private health-care through purchase of these. Within the whole NHS prescribed medication accounts for approximately a tenth of all healthcare costs, so it is clearly important that we have information about medicines, their usage, and their costs to support appropriate use of this sizeable budget.

The structure of the book looks initially at some basic information about the distribution and supply of medicines including recently introduced changes to allow wider access (Chapter 1), followed by a more detailed consideration of the overlying legal framework (Chapter 2). Then follows the very topical issue of evidence-based practice (Chapter 3) with consideration of how such information can be accessed in practice by individual prescribers (Chapter 4), patients and the public (Chapter 5). In Chapter 6, the principles of pharmacoepidemiology are introduced, with some of the topics revisited in subsequent chapters, such as performance monitoring using routine data in Chapter 7, health economics in Chapter 8 and pharmacovigilance in Chapter 9. Finally the challenges presented in accessing to best effect the enormous volume of information held across the various databases are considered (Chapter 10).

The text should be of interest to those with a clinical background but without detailed knowledge of these datasets (for example doctors, pharmacists, and new prescribers) as well as health service managers and those in academia wishing to have an overview of the key issues around medicines information.

The chapters can be read sequentially or individually. To allow the latter without irritating cross referencing to additional chapters in the book, there is inevitably a little repetition between some of the chapters. This has been kept to a minimum.

Finally my thanks go to the chapter authors, experts in their field, without whom this book would not have been possible.

Christine Bond
August 2007

About the editor

Christine Bond BPharm, FRPharmS, PhD, FFPHM has worked for Glaxo Research Laboratories, had extensive locum community pharmacist experience and is now Professor of Primary Care, and Head of the Department of General Practice and Primary Care, University of Aberdeen. She has interests in the contribution of pharmacy to effective use of medicines (prescribed and 'OTC'), drug misuse, the community pharmacist-general practitioner interface and the wider healthcare agenda. She has a grant income of over £2 million, over 150 peer-reviewed publications and is the author of two other edited books. She is part time Consultant in Pharmaceutical Public Health (NHS Grampian) and Editor of the *International Journal of Pharmacy Practice*. She is an elected member of the Scottish National Board of the Royal Pharmaceutical Society of Great Britain.

Contributors

Marion Bennie
BSc, MSc, ADCPT, MRPharmS
Chief Pharmaceutical Adviser
NHS National Services Scotland
Edinburgh

Iain Bishop
BSc, MRPharmS
Principal Pharmacist, Prescribing
Information Services Division
NHS National Services Scotland
Edinburgh

Alison Blenkinsopp
BPharm (Hons), PhD, FRPharmS
Professor of the Practice of Pharmacy
Department of Medicines Management
Keele University

Christine Bond
BPharm (Hons), MEd, PhD, FRPharmS, FFPH
Professor of Primary Care (Pharmacy)
Head of Department of General Practice
  and Primary Care
University of Aberdeen

Stephen Chapman
BSc PhD MRPhamS
Head of Department of Medicines
  Management
Keele University

Christine Clarke
PhD, MSc, BSc, FRPharmS
Medical Writer and Consultant Pharmacist
Rossendale, Lancashire

Anthony Cox BSc, MRPharmS, DipClinPharm
Teaching Fellow
Aston Pharmacy School
School of Health and Life Sciences
Aston University

Nicola Gray BSc, MRPharmS, PhD
Lecturer in Pharmacy Practice
Centre for Pharmacy, Health & Society
School of Pharmacy
University of Nottingham

Deborah Layton BSc, MRPharmS, MPhil, MSc, DipClinPharm
Research Pharmacist
Drug Safety Research Unit
Southampton

Edward J H Mallinson LLM, MPharm, FRPharmS, HonMFPH, ACPP, FRSH
Consultant in Pharmaceutical Public Health
NHS Lanarkshire
Hamilton

Stuart McTaggart BSc, MRPharmS, DipClinPharm
Senior Pharmacist
Healthcare Information Group
NHS National Services Scotland
Edinburgh

Angela Timoney MSc, MPH, ADCPT, MRPharmS
Director of Pharmacy
NHS Tayside
Dundee

Roger Walker BPharm, PhD, FRPharmS, FFPH
Professor of Pharmacy Practice
Consultant in Pharmaceutical Public Health
National Public Health Service for Wales
Cardiff

Tables and figures

Glossary

ABPI	Association of the British Pharmaceutical Industry
ACE inhibitor	angiotensin converting enzyme inhibitors
ADQ	average daily quantity
ADR	adverse drug reaction
ADROIT	Adverse Drug Reaction On-line Information Tracking
Arbuthnott Formula	a method used to calculate how to allocate central NHS funds for hospital, community health services and prescribing based on age-sex profiles, morbidity and life circumstances and remoteness
ASCOT	The Anglo-Scandinavian Cardiac Outcomes Trial
ASPP	Anonymised Single Patient Print (from ADROIT)
ASTRO-PU	age, sex, temporary resident originated prescribing unit
BMA	British Medical Association
BNF	*British National Formulary*
CDSS	clinical decision support systems
CHM	Commission on Human Medicines
CMS	Chronic Medicine Service
CI	confidence interval
CPMP	Committee for Proprietary Medicinal Products
CSM	Committee on Safety of Medicines
DAP	Drug Analysis Print (from ADROIT)
DDD	defined daily dose
dm+d	Dictionary of Medicines and Devices
DSRU	Drug Safety Research Unit
eBNF	Electronic British National Formulary
EEA	European Economic Area
EHR	electronic health record
EMEA	European Agency for the Evaluation of Medicinal Products

ENPF	extended nurse prescribers' formulary
ePACT	electronic prescribing analysis and costs
EPOS	electronic point of sale
FOI	freedom of information
Generic	not having a trademark or brand name, e.g. a generic drug
GPRD	General Practice Research Database
GSL	General Sales List medicine
ID	incidence density
IMS	a commercial provider of business intelligence and strategic consulting services for the pharmaceutical and healthcare industries
IRR	incidence density rate ratios
MEMO	Medicines Monitoring Unit, Ninewells Hospital and Medical School Dundee
MHRA	Medicines and Healthcare Products Regulatory Agency
MIMS	*Monthly Index of Medical Specialities*
MTRAC	Midlands Therapeutic Review and Advisory Committee
MUR	Medicine Use Review
NAO	National Audit Office
NHSBSA	NHS Business Services Authority
NICE	National Institute for Health and Clinical Excellence
NLH	National Library for Health
NNT	number needed to treat
NPfIT	National Programme for Information Technology
NPSA	National Patient Safety Agency
NSF	National Service Framework
OR	odds ratio
OTC	over the counter medicine
P	pharmacy only medicine
PACS	picture archiving and communication system
PACT	prescribing analysis and cost
PAGB	Proprietary Association of Great Britain
PAP	Product Analysis Print (from ADROIT)
PCT	primary care trust
PDSS	prescribing decision support system
PEM	Prescription-Event Monitoring
PMCPA	Prescription Medicines Code of Practice Authority
POM	prescription only medicine

PPA	Prescription Pricing Authority (England and Wales)
PPD	Prescription Pricing Division (Scotland)
PRODIGY	a UK national initiative to develop a computerised clinical decision support system for UK general practice. The project is funded by the NHS Executive and is based at the Sowerby Centre for Health Informatics at Newcastle
proprietary	owned by a private individual or corporation under a trademark or patent; e.g. a proprietary (branded) drug
PRR	proportional reporting ratio
PSU	prescribing support unit
PU	prescribing unit
QMAS	Quality Management and Analysis System: a national IT system which gives GP practices and primary care trusts objective evidence
QOF	Quality and Outcomes Framework: a component of the new General Medical Services contract for general practices, introduced from 1 April 2004
RAIDR	rare and iatrogenic adverse drug reactions
RAP	Reaction Analysis Print (from ADROIT)
RMC	Regional Monitoring Committee
RPSGB	Royal Pharmaceutical Society of Great Britain
RR	relative risks
SI	statutory instrument
SMC	Scottish Medicines Consortium
SmPC	Summary of Product Characteristics
SMR	Scottish Morbidity Record
SNOMED-CT®	A clinical terminology – the Systematised Nomenclature of Medicine. It is a common computerised language that will be used by all computers in the NHS to facilitate communications between healthcare professionals in clear and unambiguous terms
SPA	Scottish Prescribing Analysis
SPI	selective prostaglandin inhibition
SSRI	selective serotonin reuptake inhibitor
STAR-PU	specific therapeutic age-sex related prescribing unit
SUSAR	suspected unexpected serious adverse reaction
WHO	World Health Organization

1 Introduction

CHRISTINE BOND AND CHRISTINE CLARKE

This chapter provides a brief overview of the distribution and supply of medicines in primary and secondary care, considers how some of the routine datasets have evolved, and their uses, and concludes with consideration of some recent and imminent changes.

Overview

We are often said to live in an information age, but also to suffer from information overload. The former statement emphasises the current culture of both increasing factual knowledge about the world and the systems available to process that knowledge. These are benefits. The latter statement, on the other hand, illustrates the disadvantages and even perceived risks that are associated with this. The challenge, as always, is to learn how to maximise the benefits and minimise the risks of this situation. The title of both this book and the series within which it is published indicate support for the overall value of information. This emanates from a belief that the benefits of our information age do outweigh the disadvantages.

This book specifically looks at the information routinely available about the medicines we consume, considers the possible uses of this data, and concludes with some crystal ball gazing to consider the future. Throughout the text only medicines for human consumption are considered.

How drugs are distributed and supplied

In the UK, drugs are classified principally according to their actions and side effects into different legal classifications through the Medicines Act. These classifications control the public's access to medicines and also define how medicines are distributed and supplied. These regulatory issues are considered in more detail in Chapter 2. However, in this section we want to illustrate how the increasing use of electronic technology to streamline the process of distribution and supply per se has resulted in the accumulation of large databases of information. Whereas initially the purpose of the systems was purely one of increased efficiency in supply, the resulting datasets have now evolved into one of the biggest sources of routinely available information about the UK population's use of the medicines.

Community setting

Drugs are either classified as 'prescription only medicines' (POM), 'pharmacy only' (P) or 'General Sales List (GSL) medicines'.

In the community setting, the traditional route of supply of 'prescription only medicines' to the public has been if a doctor (general practitioner), or for a limited range of drugs a dentist, has prescribed them. There are increasingly changes in this model but these are described later, and here we will just focus on the traditional model. The mechanism is that after the doctor has written the prescription, it is then taken to a community pharmacist for the drugs to be dispensed from stock held by the pharmacist. The cost of the drugs is reimbursed to the pharmacist, by the UK Government, through the Prescription Pricing Authority in England and Wales and the Prescription Pricing Division in Scotland. In order to do this all prescription forms, once the medicines have been dispensed by the pharmacist, are returned to a central point, and the data entered onto a national computer. What was not particularly appreciated when the system was introduced was that the dataset of dispensed medicines, linked to both doctors and pharmacists, could be used for a range of interesting retrospective analyses of trends in drug use and patterns of morbidity. Thus as systems have been reviewed and refined this aspect of their functionality has been considered in its own right, and developed to improve the accuracy and validity of the datasets. This is discussed in more detail in Chapter 7.

Likewise within general practices, computing technology was originally introduced to support appointment procedures and other administrative functions, such as the generation of repeat prescriptions. Indeed the acronym of the main system in use in Scotland is GPASS which stands for General Practice Administration System Scotland. Other commercially available and widely used systems include EMIS, VISION, VAMP and TORIX. Once small amounts of prescribing data, even only repeat prescribing, became part of the dataset the potential of the system as a source of information was again quickly recognised. Unlike the dispensed dataset required for the reimbursement and remuneration of community pharmacists the completeness of the data has often been questioned. This is because it depends on GPs voluntarily using it due to its increased working efficiency compared to traditional paper-based systems. Increasingly, the value of the system has been recognised as a source of Health Service statistics. GPs have become more willing to use the system for a wider range of activities, and now not only repeat but also acute prescribing is done largely through the computer, supported by a range of decision support software. When the ultimate main purpose of a dataset is not that which was originally intended, there will naturally be aspects that need to be amended and this has happened progressively with software upgrades which have continually become more clinical in their content and focus, whilst supporting the administrative functions of the practice with increased efficiency. This is discussed in more detail in some of the chapters that follow.

Recent changes to the Medicines Act have enabled the prescription of some 'POM' medicines not just by medical practitioners but by a range of other specially trained and accredited healthcare professionals such as nurses, pharmacists and chiropodists, for certain specified conditions. This deregulation of NHS supply is likely to expand, particularly for nurses and pharmacists, to include most *BNF* medicines. Maintaining a comprehensive record of prescribed medicines at individual patient level will become increasingly challenging. These changes and their implications for medicines information are discussed in more detail in Chapter 10.

At the moment, and with individual patient consent, community pharmacists keep computerised records of the prescriptions they have dispensed, building up an historical record of patients' drug regimens. These records are known as PMRs (Patient Medication Records). Again completeness of data is an issue because patients are allowed in theory to take a prescription anywhere to be dispensed. Although evidence suggests that 80–90% of patients always use the same pharmacy, adherence to this historical right challenges the comprehensiveness of the dataset. So for the moment, other than for sharing of patient information between individual pharmacy members of a multiple organisation, pharmacy held data is probably of greatest value at an individual patient level.

We shall now consider the non-prescription medicines which are distributed via community pharmacists. As noted above this group includes both those medicinal products restricted by regulations to sale through community pharmacists (the P medicines), and those medicines free of any regulatory restrictions (the General Sales List medicines) under the Medicines Act. This group of medicines is steadily increasing in both number and potency at the present time as the UK Government pursues its policy of increasing access to medicines and encouraging self-care and self-responsibility in the management of minor and self-limiting conditions. This is again discussed in more detail in Chapter 10. One of the problems with this is that if medicines are not going through the traditional prescribed route their usage is not captured routinely by either of the IT systems mentioned above. However, statistics are available on the quantities supplied to community pharmacies through wholesalers and it can be assumed that this closely follows supply. Thus collation of this data, as is done by a range of commercial companies such as IMS, can usefully show trends in OTC (over the counter) medicines use. Likewise individual pharmacies using EPOS systems (electronic point of sale) for stock control can produce statistics for their own sales volumes.

Finally there is least information on those drugs distributed not just through community pharmacies but also through other general sales outlets. This includes a range of commercial settings including petrol stations, corner shops and supermarkets. Because of the diverse range of settings there is no easy or opportunistic way to capture routine statistics on their supply and distribution. The limitations and concerns arising from this are again detailed more in Chapter 10.

Hospital settings

In the hospital setting, medicines are prescribed by doctors and supplied by the hospital pharmacy department. On some occasions supplies are made to named patients but on many occasions the medicines are issued by nurses from supplies held on the ward known as 'ward stock'.

Computerised pharmacy stock control systems have been in use for more than 20 years. Although they were originally developed as a means of streamlining the complex ordering processes needed to manage several thousand lines of goods with variable usage patterns, it soon became clear that valuable data on patterns of usage and expenditure were being amassed. In the first instance this data was only available at hospital level. However, where computerised records of issues of medicines to wards and departments were also made, and in some cases to specialties or individual patients, more detailed datasets became available. Medicines dispensed on discharge and those supplied to outpatients (in England and Wales) have almost always been recorded individually, providing another rich source of data.

The introduction of computerised prescribing systems has created opportunities to capture useful data more easily. It is no longer necessary for pharmacy staff to transcribe prescription information from paper documents into pharmacy stock control systems. Details of the prescriber are captured when he or she logs in and prescription data is captured when written. Electronic linkage between stock control and prescribing systems ensures that there is an electronic audit trail from wholesaler to patient. Linked electronic medicines administration systems will complete the picture.

The use of this information has gone through several stages as the information technology has developed. Pharmacy managers have been able to compare drug usage and expenditure patterns between consultants and specialties and also within specialties over time. Such reports have been used extensively in cost-containment initiatives. When more detailed datasets became available pharmacists and clinicians were able to work together to monitor compliance with prescribing guidelines for specific products and to identify potential problems with high-risk medicines.

We have already had glimpses in isolated projects of the types of things that might be possible in future. The development of individual electronic health records, accessible throughout the NHS, and the underpinning technologies will enable complete records of individual drug treatment to be reviewed and monitored. At a population level it will mean that medicine use and expenditure can be linked to clinical outcomes.

Value and use of routine data for managers, prescribers and patients/medicine takers

Managers

It is of worldwide concern, and no less so in the UK than other developed countries, that the cost of our prescribed medicines is increasing year on year. Although the UK spends less per head of the population on prescribed medicine than many other countries, nonetheless for many years the total sum has been approximately 10% of the total NHS budget. In more recent years this has slowly increased to 11%. In primary care the cost of drugs dispensed is approximately 60% of all NHS costs – that is more than all the other costs of salaries, premises, referrals and tests put together. Thus at a time when the NHS is making hard decisions about the affordability of other innovations in healthcare – be they other new drugs, new techniques or merely more staff – even small percentage reductions in drug expenditure could generate significant savings enabling other innovations to be introduced.

It is therefore not surprising that healthcare managers are particularly interested in information on prescribing costs such as is generated by the systems described above. These can be used to monitor trends in the use of medicines; for example, to define the market penetration of new drugs or to assess the quality of an individual doctor's prescribing. An illustration of the latter would be, for example, in monitoring good antibiotic prescribing, such as looking at the ratio of co-amoxiclav to co-amoxiclav plus amoxicillin. The point of this ratio is that the two drugs would be commonly prescribed for the same condition, but amoxicillin would be the drug of choice on the basis of both cost and safety. Similar ratios and performance indicators have been derived for a whole range of therapeutic conditions.

This sort of information is used to target poor prescribers at doctor level, or poor practices at a locality level, or poor primary care organisations at a national level. After adjusting for known sources of variability such as the age and sex of the population, amazing differences can still emerge between prescribers which are unexplained. These differences have been the source of many research projects and much speculation. For example, consideration of the adjusted spend per head of the population in primary care by different health board areas of Scotland is known to vary considerably. What is interesting to managers is that increased spending does not translate into equivalently improved health across different areas. Thus the challenge is to make sure that prescribers use drugs in a cost effective and clinically effective way.

Prescribers

It is also of course important for individual prescribers to get feedback on their actual prescribing practice. The fallacies of retrospective self-reporting of behaviours are well documented. Anecdotally doctors are known to be totally confident that they never prescribe a particular drug, perhaps one which is rather new and costly when there are cheaper established generic products available. Inevitably when incontrovertible individual prescribing feedback is looked at they are surprised. Support for GPs in interpreting the sometimes unfriendly reporting styles of computerised feedback is often provided by pharmacist prescribing advisers who are trained in the interpretation of the statistics and in agreeing on strategies for behavioural change with the GPs.

This analysis of personal prescribing is a good vehicle for targeted individual campaigns which contribute to area-wide initiatives in reducing drug costs, or improving prescribing. For example, at the moment there are general concerns about antibiotic resistance. Within this area there are particular concerns such as overuse of individual antibiotics, for example co-amoxiclav instead of amoxicillin (see earlier reference to this), or use of third generation cephalosporins for routine and often minor infections, instead of symptomatic treatment, or older antibiotics as first line therapy. Such behaviours can readily be monitored with the prescribing datasets we have already described. This will be covered more in Chapter 7.

Patients and medicine takers

Those that take medicines also need information. The medical administration systems not only evolved into prescribing databases, but also nearly all general practices in the UK now hold patient medical records on computerised files. Thus it is increasingly easy for prescribers to cross-check an individual's medical and drug history before prescribing additional therapy, thus reducing the chances of prescribing a contraindicated drug or causing a drug–drug interaction.

The collation of data on populations also enables rare and sometimes fatal events to be identified, as is described in Chapter 9. Whilst spontaneous reporting is the source of data for the main regulatory database held by the MHRA, the Yellow Card system, dedicated exercises make use of linkage across the datasets described above. For example, the Tayside based MEMO unit has developed an internationally recognised expertise in data linkage across primary and secondary care and including pharmacy data.

Drug formularies

There are many thousands of active drug entities, and even more individual products, when different combinations of drugs, and different branded preparations of the same drugs, are considered.

Compendia listing all available products have always been a source of invaluable knowledge to those making recommendations to patients for a POM, P or GSL medicine.

Early national formularies in the UK include the *British National Formulary* (BNF), a publication produced jointly by the Royal Pharmaceutical Society of Great Britain (RPSGB), and the British Medical Association (BMA). This was first published as the *National Formulary* in 1949 and included fewer than 300 entries, many of which were formulae for the preparation of a mixture or ointment from its basic ingredients. The quality of, and specification for, the basic ingredients were defined in the *British Pharmacopoeia*, first published in 1864 by the General Council of Medical Education and Registration in the UK, and its companion volume the *British Pharmaceutical Codex* (first published by Direction of the Council of the Pharmaceutical Society of Great Britain in 1907). Both of these are still in print as later editions although transformed in appearance, content and frequency of publication.

The current *BNF*, issue 54, now lists many hundreds of products and includes invaluable information on indications, contraindications and preferred therapies, as well as providing information on nurse and dental formularies, drug interactions, and much other useful information for prescribers. Other useful texts providing information on drugs include the *Martindale Extra Pharmacopoeia*, the *United States Pharmacopoeia*, and the *Merck Index*.

As the numbers of drugs and products has escalated, it has been widely recognised that in order to help doctors prescribe both clinically and cost effectively, a smaller personal formulary is required. For a GP a list of 150–200 drugs should be sufficient to treat all but the very rare conditions. This restricted list makes it more likely that the prescriber can be familiar with the costs and benefits of individual drugs. Initially practice formularies were seen as the way forward, with some acknowledgement that a large part of their value was in the compilation process as much as in the use.

Likewise, hospitals also developed formularies to promote preferred products, control prescribing by hospital staff, and allow more limited stocks to be maintained.

Most recently the individual practice formularies and hospital formularies have been combined into area wide or 'joint' formularies. The advantages of this are that patients moving from one care setting to another, as occurs at admission to or discharge from hospital, are more likely to get continuity of treatment.

The skills in agreeing on formulary content have also developed and great care and expertise is now required to ensure drugs listed are clinically and cost effective. This topic of evidence-based medicine and the trend for national approaches and guidance is addressed more in Chapter 3.

Consideration of some future developments

Future developments centre around changes in the distribution and supply of medicine and IT developments. They are summarised in this chapter and described in more detail in Chapter 10.

Changes in the distribution and supply of medicines

As noted above there are concerns within healthcare about the ever-increasing cost of NHS drugs and the need to meet patients' ever-increasing demands for access to healthcare. One of the ways of addressing the former has been to remove drugs from prescription, only supply to pharmacy availability and ultimately general sale. This means, in lay terms, that the public can buy an increasing range of drugs with which to self-medicate, without recourse to a doctor. Additionally the range of professionals able to prescribe is also increasing through the use of Patient Group Directions, Direct Supply Projects, supplementary and independent prescribing.

Independent prescribing for nurses was first introduced in 1994 on a pilot basis, initially based on a very limited formulary of products. This has subsequently been extended significantly with an accredited 'advanced' nurse prescriber now able to prescribe from an extended nurse prescribers' formulary (ENPF). Most recently further legislative changes have authorised nurses to prescribe any drug for any condition, as long as they operate within their own self-determined level of professional competence. At the same time, independent prescribing by pharmacists will also be allowed. Pharmacists and nurses prescribing under these new regulations will need to undergo additional, but relatively minimal, training, above and beyond their core professional qualification. It is anticipated that this might just be an interim arrangement and that ultimately this training will be incorporated into undergraduate curricula.

New community pharmacy contracts being introduced in England, Wales and Scotland recognise these new routes of supply and changed roles for pharmacy. In England and Wales, the pharmacy contract is in three tiers. The basic tier which all pharmacists will deliver does not include a direct supply route in contrast to Scotland where there are four core services: chronic medicine service which will encompass supplementary prescribing, acute medicine services which is the traditional dispensing role, minor ailment services which encompass the direct supply schemes, and public health services. Additional locally negotiated services in public health may well use patient group directions for supply of, for example, smoking cessation products or emergency hormonal contraception.

The implication of these changes is that medicines, some of them potent, will be supplied by a new range of professionals. Whilst record keeping and audit trails will be maintained, there will no longer be a single database to inform us of usage.

Enhanced IT

It is almost inconceivable when so much of commerce depends on electronic data interchange, and compatibility of different systems, and different levels of read and write access to common datasets, that the NHS still depends on a multiplicity of systems which have developed in parallel, and cannot be used in an integrated way.

Therefore the changes in supply and distribution of drugs described in the previous section potentially could limit the comprehensiveness and therefore value of the databases we currently use to inform our use of medicines. Whilst record keeping is central to all the new supply routes there is at the moment no single record which can hold all the information, thus reducing the opportunity for early detection/ avoidance of contraindicated drug use, or drug interactions, or the linking of adverse drug reactions and side effects to presentation of new symptoms. Similarly there is currently no link, even within the medical fraternity, for the sharing of medical information across primary and secondary care.

There are signs that all of this is changing, but as with many IT projects, progress in implementation is slow, whilst advances in technology are accelerating, quickly rendering state of the art software and hardware redundant. Meanwhile capital costs are high, therefore decision making has huge implications.

Nonetheless, progress on linking primary care general practice and hospital systems is moving. In primary care it may soon be possible for any doctor to access a patient's record; for example, from a different geographical area than their home base.

Similarly community pharmacists are slowly being connected to the NHS net; whilst initially this will primarily be used for email communications and electronic transmission of prescription data from general practitioner to community pharmacist, the linkage could ultimately facilitate two-way access to medical records. This might be used, for example, so that the community pharmacist could check a patient's medical record before making a new prescribing decision, either by supplementary prescribing, or direct supply, or an OTC sale, and then 'write' information back to the record once the supply had been made, thus maintaining the comprehensiveness of the dataset. Alternatively unique patient identifiers could be used to ensure all data relating to a singe patient could be linked. Research shows that there may be barriers to be overcome, as we move towards such an integrated system. For example, there will be issues of agreeing relative professional accountabilities, and ensuring patient confidentiality. None of these is insurmountable, and should not be used as reasons for failing to progress.

Conclusion

In conclusion this chapter has set the scene for the rest of this volume. It has highlighted the wide range of drugs available, and outlined their supply routes, the datasets, and their uses. Medicine distribution and supply is undergoing radical change at a time when information of medicine usage is of increasing value to a range of stakeholders. It is up to everyone to work together to maintain the benefit of a comprehensive database whilst deregulation of medicines supply provides safe and convenient public access. All of these are returned to in more detail in succeeding chapters.

2 Regulatory issues

EDWARD MALLINSON

This chapter briefly reviews some key issues in the history of drug regulation, then summarises the main regulations which now affect medicines, their distribution and supply.

Introduction

The regulation and control of medicinal products has long been known. The first pharmacopoeia was produced in Italy as long ago as 1498 with the first approved list of drugs in a *London Pharmacopoeia* in 1618. Others followed in Scotland in 1699 (the *Edinburgh Pharmacopoeia*) and Ireland in 1807 (the *Dublin Pharmacopoeia*) and the first *British Pharmacopoeia* was published in 1864.

The Pharmaceutical Society of Great Britain (now the Royal Pharmaceutical Society) was formed in 1841 by a group of London chemists and druggists with a view to initiating uniformity within the profession. The Society was granted a Royal charter in 1843 and became the regulatory body for pharmacists in 1933 as a result of the Pharmacy & Poisons Act.[1]

Licensing of medicinal products within the UK was not introduced until 1925 with the enactment of the Therapeutic Substances Act.[2] This, however, only covered 'the regulation of manufacture, sale and importation of vaccines, sera and other therapeutic substances', the purity or potency of which cannot adequately be tested by chemical means.[3] The schedule outlining those products covered by the Act contained only four sections.[4] The discovery and use of anti-microbial agents such as penicillin resulted in two further Acts of Parliament[5,6] in 1947 and 1953. These three were finally repealed in 1956 and replaced with an updated Therapeutic Substances Act.[7]

The main stimulus for modern day licensing and control of medicines came in the early 1960s as a direct result of the thalidomide tragedy. Thalidomide was first marketed in Germany in 1959 as a sedative. In the early years of its use it appeared to be particularly safe and had few if any side effects. It was widely prescribed to pregnant women to combat 'morning sickness' and was marketed worldwide, both on prescription and equally 'over the counter' in pharmacies. However, in December 1961, Dr WG McBride, an Australian obstetrician and gynaecologist, published a letter in the *Lancet*[8] reporting congenital abnormalities in 1.5% of babies born to mothers who had taken the drug during pregnancy and asking if others had encountered similar occurrences. The manufacturers, the Distillers Company (Biochemicals) Limited, had been alerted to other reports and the drug was withdrawn from the market, pending further investigation, in November 1961.

What followed was to change the course of pharmaceutical manufacture forever. In 1963 the UK government responded by forming the Committee on Safety of Drugs (the Dunlop Committee) under the chairmanship of Sir Derek Dunlop. This committee had no legal power but entered into voluntary arrangements with the Association of British Pharmaceutical Industry (ABPI). This was the first attempt to control the manufacture and testing of medicines in the UK.

The first piece of legislation to result from the work of the committee was the Medicines Act[9] which received Royal Assent on 25 October 1968; however, it did not come into force until 1971 nearly 10 years after Dr McBride published his findings on thalidomide.

The Medicines Act

The Medicines Act is 165 pages in length, has 136 sections and eight schedules and is in eight parts.

Part I   Administration
       This section describes the responsibilities of Ministers and the establishment and functions of the Medicines Commission and its committees.

Part II   Licences and Certificates relating to Medicinal Products
           This section gives detail of the licensing authority and
           provisions dealing with medicinal products, their manu-
           facturing and wholesaling. It also covers exemptions,
           suspension, revocation and variation of licences, together
           with information relating to clinical trials and medicated
           animal feeds.

Part III   Provisions relating to dealings with Medicinal Products
           This section covers provisions relating to the sale and supply
           of medicinal products, together with the appropriate exemp-
           tions and restrictions.

Part IV   Pharmacies
           This section covers the criteria for conducting a lawful retail
           pharmacy business, the registration of retail pharmacies,
           the use of restricted titles and the removal of premises from
           the register.

Part V   Containers, Packages, and Identification of Medicinal
           Products
           This section deals with the law relating to the packaging of
           medicinal products and leaflets included with medicines.

Part VI   Promotion of sales of Medicinal Products
           This section deals with the law relating to the advertising of
           medicinal products and its regulation.

Part VII   British Pharmacopoeia and other publications.

Part VIII Miscellaneous and Supplemental Provisions
           This section covers a range of issues relating mainly to
           enforcement of the Act and Regulations in each of the four
           home countries, including definition of offences, interpreta-
           tion of terms used within the Act and financial provisions.

The parts of most relevance are Part II, Part III and Part VI.

Medicines classification

Medicines are classified in three categories in the UK:

- prescription only medicines (POM)
- pharmacy medicines (P)
- General Sales List (GSL) medicines.

Prescription only medicines are only available to the general public following the dispensing of a prescription written by an authorised prescriber. In the past this has been either a doctor or a dentist. However, in 1998 a limited number of specially trained nurses was authorised to prescribe drugs listed in the *Nurse Prescribers Formulary*.[10] These nurses were drawn from District Nurses, Health Visitors and some Practice Nurses. The Health and Social Care Act extended the group of professionals who are allowed to prescribe and clauses in the Act enable Ministers to introduce new types of prescriber, who will be responsible for the continuing care of patients who have already been clinically assessed by a doctor.[11] Further information about the supply and administration of medicines will be covered in the section on Patient Group Directions later in this chapter, and is also referred to again in Chapter 10.

Pharmacy medicines do not require a written prescription by an authorised prescriber (see above), although this does not preclude them from being prescribed, but are only available for sale from a community pharmacy under the supervision of a registered pharmacist. The Act defines a community pharmacy as a 'registered pharmacy'.[12] The restriction on the advertising of such medicines will be discussed later in this chapter.

General Sales List medicines are defined as '(medicinal) products which in their (appropriate Minister's) opinion can, with reasonable safety, be sold or supplied otherwise than by, or under the supervision of, a pharmacist'. Many medicines in this category can be found on supermarket shelves or in shops on garage forecourts.

Medicines in each of the above categories are issued with 'marketing authorisations' or 'product licences' by the Medicines and Healthcare Products Regulatory Agency (MHRA) (previously known as the Medicines Control Agency (MCA)) or by the European Agency for the Evaluation of Medicinal Products (EMEA). The scope of the powers of these licensing bodies is laid down in Regulations.[13] In reaching a decision on whether or not to grant a licence the MHRA:

... shall in particular take into consideration:

(a) the safety of medicinal products of each description to which the application relates;
(b) the efficacy of medicinal products of each such description for the purposes for which the products are proposed to be administered; and
(c) the quality of medicinal products of each such description, according to the specification and the method or proposed method of manufacture of the products, and the provisions proposed for securing that the products as sold or supplied will be of that quality.[14]

Applying for a licence

Applications for a marketing authorisation (previously known as a product licence) for new active substances, new delivery systems and the first generic version of an established medicinal product are automatically referred to the main advisory body for the evaluation of human medicines, namely the Committee on Safety of Medicines (CSM). If an authorisation is granted, following scrutiny of a vast amount of data on the product's quality, safety and efficacy, it is normal for it be restricted for use under medical supervision and classified as a prescription only medicine (POM).

If, after several years of experience of its use, the manufacture can convince the MHRA that the product is safe enough for use under pharmacist supervision they can apply to have the product reclassified as a P medicine. This change is not automatic and although the procedures for reclassification were simplified in April 2002 most applications still take between five and seven months to be processed. It is time consuming and expensive and, therefore, if the initiative has come from the industry as opposed to the professional bodies, subsequent marketing will be used to optimise sales, ensure a viable product and an adequate return on investment. This includes direct advertising to the public which can lead to problems in practice, because it raises patient expectations and can create inappropriate demand for a product. The advertising is regulated by the industry under the auspices of the Proprietary Association of Great Britain (PAGB), and standards have recently been raised to come into line with the 1992 European Pharmaceutical Advertising Directive.

Advertising of medicinal products

The advertising of medicinal products is controlled by the Medicines Act 1968 and the Regulation made under it. These take cognisance of EEC directives which have been issued in the years following 1968. In addition the Association of the British Pharmaceutical Industry (ABPI) and the Proprietary Association of Great Britain each have Codes of Practice [15, 16, 17] which supplement the legislation.

The first legal restrictions on the advertising of medicinal products were introduced in the Venereal Diseases Act 1917 in section 2 namely:

> 2. – (2) on or after the first day of November nineteen hundred and seventeen a person shall not hold out or recommend to the public by any notice or advertisement, or by any written or printed papers or handbills, or by any label or words written or printed, affixed to or delivered with, any packet, box, bottle, phial, or any other enclosure containing the same, any pills, capsules, powders, lozenges, tinctures, potions, cordials, electuaries, plaisters, unguents, salves, ointments, drops, lotions, oils, spirits, medicated herbs and waters, chemical and officinal preparations whatsoever, to be used or applied externally or internally as medicines or medicaments for the prevention, cure, or relief of any venereal disease:
>
> Provided that nothing in this section shall apply to any advertisement, notification, announcement, recommendation, or holding out made or published by any local or public authority or made or published with the sanction of the Local Government Board, or in Scotland and Ireland the Local Government Board for Scotland and Ireland respectively, or to any publication sent only to duly qualified medical practitioners or to wholesale or retail chemists for the purposes of their business.

Present day control over the advertising of medicinal products is covered by:
- The Medicines Act 1968 part VI
- The Trades Descriptions Act 1968
- Control of Misleading Advertisements Act 1988,

the following EC Directives:
- 84/450/EEC   Misleading Advertisements
- 89/552/EEC   Television Advertisements
- 92/28/EEC   Advertising of medicinal products for human use,

and the Code of Practice for the Pharmaceutical Industry 2006 produced by the Prescription Medicines Code of Practice Authority (PMCPA) together with the Code of Advertising Practice for Over-the-Counter Medicines produced by the Proprietary Association of Great Britain.

In addition the standard provisions of the product licence control advertising. If these are not complied with, the product licence can be revoked.

The legislation draws a distinction between 'advertisement' and 'representation'.

The former includes:

> every form of advertising, whether in a publication, or by display of any notice, or by means of any catalogue, price list, letter (whether circular or addressed to a particular person) or other document, or by words inscribed on any article, or by the exhibition of a photograph or a cinematograph film, or by way of sound recording, sound broadcasting or television, or in any other way.[18]

The latter means:

> any statement or undertaking (whether constituting a condition or a warranty or not) which consists of spoken words other than words broadcast by sound recording, sound broadcasting or television, or forming part of a sound recording or embodied in a cinematograph film soundtrack.[19]

The Regulations[20] controlling the advertising of medicinal products to healthcare professionals (i.e. advertisements wholly or mainly directed at persons qualified to prescribe or supply relevant medicinal products)[21] incorporate the EEC Directive (92/28/EEC) and prevent any person issuing an advertisement unless it contains the following information:

- the licence number of the product
- the name and address of the marketing organisation holder
- the classification of the product (POM, P, or GSL)
- the name of the product
- a list of the active ingredients
- the licensed indications

- a short summary of the 'summary of product characteristics' (SPC).

An abbreviated advertisement is one other than a loose insert (i.e., it is part of a professional publication) which does not exceed 420 square centimetres in area and should contain the following:
- the product name (either proprietary or non-proprietary)
- a list of the active ingredients
- the name and address of the product licence holder
- words indicating that further information is available on the SPC.

The above do not extend to 'promotional aids' if the advertisement consists only of the name of the product and is intended to be merely an 'aide memoire'.

The regulations also cover hospitality and inducements. Here the licence holder or his or her representative may not offer any gift, monetary advantage or benefit in kind to healthcare professionals unless it is inexpensive and relevant to the practice of medicine or pharmacy. The offer of hospitality to healthcare professionals must be purely for professional or scientific purposes. It must be of a reasonable level and subordinate to the main purpose of the meeting.

The regulations governing the advertisement of medicinal products to the general public are included in SI 1994 No.1932 and state that no advertisement should be issued in connection with:
- a controlled drug (Regulation 8)
- a prescription-only medicine for human use (Regulation 7)
- an abortifacient (Regulation 6)
- treatment, prevention and diagnosis of certain diseases (Regulation 6).

The advert should not contain information which is laid down in Regulation 9. In particular it should not contain guarantees of the efficacy of the product or an indication that a person's health may be enhanced by taking the product.

Very few cases have come before the Courts relating to breaches of the Medicines Act and its Regulations. In 1986 Roussel Laboratories, a pharmaceutical company and its Medical Director, Dr Christopher Good, were convicted at the Central Criminal Court of offences under section 93 of the Medicines Act 1968. They were convicted of issuing a false and misleading advertisement relating to a medicinal product, Surgam®, a non-steroidal anti-inflammatory drug (NSAID), which was published in several editions of the *British Medical Journal* during March, April and May of 1983. The advertisement led the reader to believe that the gastric side effects, which are well known in other NSAIDs, of this product were less, due to selective prostaglandin inhibition (SPI). Research had previously shown no difference in the SPI of Surgam® (their product) and Indocid® (indomethacin), another NSAID.[22] It was alleged that the advertisement 'was likely to mislead as to the nature or quality of the product'. The subsequent appeal of 20 May 1988 was dismissed.[23] In their judgement Watkins LJ, Hollings and Peter Palin J held that:

- 'quality' in section 93 (7) was not confined to 'commercial quality or grade' and included character, characteristics and attributes of the product
- the word 'Quality' was not to receive the restricted meaning it had been given in the case law on section 2 (1) Food & Drugs Act 1955[24]
- the Jury had to look at the advertisement *as a whole* [my emphasis], taking into account that the target reader was a General Practitioner.

Peter Palin J added:

> In future prosecutions under this section it is desirable in the interests of everyone concerned that the particulars of the offence should contain the word or words relied upon with specific reference to s 93(7)(b), that is to say whether the likelihood of someone being misled by the advertisement is alleged to be as one or more, specifying which, of the words, 'nature, quality, uses or effects'.

It should be noted that the case took a considerable time to get to Court and resulted in a large fine for the company (which, it could be argued, was probably outweighed by the revenue received from sales of the product as a result of the advertisement).

The main control of advertising of medicines is carried out by the ABPI and PAGB using their respective Codes of Conduct.

The former regulates its members using the Prescription Medicines Code of Practice Authority (PMCPA). The Chairman is legally qualified and the committee meets every six weeks. It is responsible for the administration of the Code of Practice for the Pharmaceutical

Industry including the provision of advice, guidance and training on the Code. It is also responsible for the conciliation between companies when requested to do so and for scrutinising journal advertising on a regular basis.[25] The Authority also administers the complaints procedure by which complaints made under the Code are considered by the Code of Practice Panel and, where required, by the Code of Practice Appeal Board.[26]

The Code applies to the promotion of medicines to members of the UK (including the Channel Islands and the Isle of Man) health professions and to appropriate administrative staff and to information made available to the general public about medicines so promoted.[27]

When the Panel finds that there has been a breach of the Code, the company concerned is so advised and given reasons for the decision. The company is given 10 working days to provide the Panel with a written undertaking that the promotional activity will cease immediately and that all possible steps will be taken to avoid a similar breach in the future. The company must also pay, within 20 working days, an administrative charge based on the number of matters ruled in breach of the Code.[28]

In June 1988 The Code of Practice Committee ruled against Professional Counselling Aids Limited and were taken to Court by the latter.[29] It was argued by the company that the decision of the committee was unreasonable[30] and that the committee was subject to Judicial Review. Mr Justice Popplewell ruled that the committee's decision, although one which he would not have necessarily endorsed, was not one which the court could reverse. However, on the question of jurisdiction he ruled, with great reluctance, that the Court did have jurisdiction in such cases. He indicated that the test to be applied was: 'were the proceedings of the committee purely domestic or was there a public duty involved?' Thus the deliberations of the Code of Practice Committee are set in the context of the courts.

In May 1997, *The Sunday Times* reported that Lagap Pharmaceuticals, a pharmaceutical company, had offered gift vouchers to pharmacists, valid in various stores, in return for the purchase of medicines. A similar allegation was made against Approved Prescription Services, another company. Both cases were referred to the PMCPA. Both companies defended the scheme by stating that:

> vouchers were only available as an alternative to discounts and thus were not gifts or inducements which are prohibited under the code,

but were matters related to prices, margins and discounts, which do not come under the code. The companies also argued that as the schemes were directed at Pharmacists, and not doctors, they could not be said to influence medication received by patients.[31]

The PMCPA panel ruled that such offers were not related to prices, margins or discounts and thus were prohibited gifts and inducements to health professionals. This breached the ABPI code of advertising practice clause 18.1 which states:

> No gift, benefit in kind or pecuniary advantage shall be offered or given to members of the health professions or to administrative staff as an inducement to prescribe, supply, administer or buy any medicine . . .

The PAGB vets advertisements prior to publication, unlike the PMCPA. The Association's conditions of membership require its members to submit the following material relevant to labelling, packaging, advertising and promotion of their products to the public:

- TV and radio commercials
- packaging – cartons and other containers
- labels
- leaflets
- booklets
- point of sale material
- posters
- print advertisements (for use in newspaper, magazines etc.)
- aerial promotions
- direct mail
- sales promotion material including reader write-in offers.

It is therefore understandable that this has assisted its members in maintaining a high level of compliance with both the statutory and voluntary requirements.

It can be seen from the foregoing that the pharmaceutical industry attempts to regulate the advertising of medicines with particular vigour and only when this self-regulation fails does it have recourse to the Courts. In all only three cases have come before the Courts in recent years which indicates that self-regulation is effective. However, it could be argued that once an advert has appeared then the message it has communicated is difficult to reverse in the minds of the recipient audience. For this reason the PAGB system of vetting adverts pre-publication is to be commended. The ultimate sanction under the Regulations is the withdrawal of the product licence and no pharmaceutical company can afford to risk this happening to it.

Supply and administration

Prescription only medicines can only be supplied or administered 'in accordance with a prescription supplied by an appropriate practitioner'.[32] Up until the introduction of Supplementary Prescribing, and Patient Group Directions, this meant only a doctor, dentist, veterinary surgeon or veterinary practitioner (the latter two for animal medicines only).

Patient Group Directions

In August 2000, following wide consultation exemption was granted in the situation where the administration or supply was undertaken in accordance with a Patient Group Direction (PGD).[33]

PGDs allow supply or administration of a prescription only medicine by specified NHS bodies and specified individuals. They must be:
- written
- signed by a doctor or dentist and a pharmacist
- signed by a representative of the specified body.

They must also:
- be in effect at the time of the supply
- contain certain particulars
- be signed by the authorised persons, carried out by the named practitioner and relate to a licensed medicine or registered homeopathic medicine.

Initially PGDs applied only to the National Health Service; however, in 2003 regulations were made allowing their use in special healthcare establishments provided through the private, charitable or voluntary sectors.[34]

In all cases the PGD should include the following:[35]
- the name of the business to which the direction applies
- the date the direction comes into force and the date it expires
- a description of the medicine(s) to which the direction applies

- class of health professional who may supply or administer the medicine
- signature of a doctor or dentist, as appropriate, and a pharmacist
- signature by an appropriate organisation
- the clinical condition or situation to which the direction applies
- a description of those patients excluded from treatment under the direction
- a description of the circumstances in which further advice should be sought from a doctor (or dentist, as appropriate) and arrangements for referral
- details of appropriate dosage and maximum total dosage, quantity, pharmaceutical form and strength, route and frequency of administration, and minimum or maximum period over which the medicine should be administered
- relevant warnings, including potential adverse reactions
- details of any necessary follow-up action and the circumstances
- a statement of the records to be kept for audit purposes.

It should be borne in mind, however, that a person supplying or administering medicines under the terms of a PGD is *not* prescribing in a strict legal sense.

Supplementary prescribing

Supplementary prescribing is a *'voluntary partnership between an independent prescriber (a doctor or dentist) and a supplementary prescriber to implement an agreed patient-specific Clinical Management Plan with the patient's agreement'*.[36]

Supplementary prescribers are defined as:

a. a first level nurse;
b. a pharmacist;
c. a registered midwife;
d. a person whose name is registered in part of the register maintained by the Health Professions Council in pursuant of article 5 of the Health Professions Order 2001 relating to:
   i. chiropodists and podiatrists;
   ii. physiotherapists; or
   iii. radiographers; diagnostic or therapeutic; or
e. a registered optometrist.[37]

The first stage in the process is the formulation of the patient's clinical management plan. Once this is agreed to by all parties, the supplementary prescriber is empowered to prescribe any medicine referred to in the plan for that patient. There is no formulary or restricted list. Further information on supplementary prescribing can be found in *Medicines Matters* published by the Department of Health.[38]

Conclusion

Medicines are potent products, the use of which is highly regulated in the interests of patients. Recently some relaxations in supply have been introduced, recognising the need to improve patient convenience, and utilise more fully the skills of a wider range of highly trained healthcare professionals. The wider range of options around access to medicines also reflects societal changes around the deregulation of professions, and changing dynamics in professional-client relationships. However, against this backdrop patient safety remains paramount, and changes, particularly in medicines classification, are always under review. The role of pharmacovigilance in this regard is covered in Chapter 9.

References

1. The Pharmacy and Poisons Act, 1933; ch 25 part 1.
2. The Therapeutic Substances Act, 1925; ch 60.
3. Ibid. s(1).
4. Ibid. Schedule.
5. The Penicillin Act, 1947; ch 29.
6. The Therapeutic Substances (Prevention of Misuse) Act, 1953; ch 32.
7. The Therapeutic Substances Act, 1956; ch 25.
8. McBride WG. *The Lancet* 1961; **16 December**: 1358.
9. The Medicines Act, 1968; ch 67.
10. *British National Formulary* **48**; 834–41.
11. Health and Social Services Act, 2001; ch 15 s63.
12. Ibid. s74(1).
13. The Medicines for Human Use (Marketing Authorisation etc.) Regulations, 1994 (SI 1994 No 3144).
14. The Medicines Act, 1968; ch 67 s19(1).
15. 'Code of Practice for the Pharmaceutical Industry, 1998'; Prescription Medicines Code of Practice Authority.
16. 'Code of Standards of Advertising Practice for Over-the-Counter Medicines', 1994.

17. 'Code of Standards for Advertising Over-the-Counter Medicines to Health Professionals and the Retail Trade', 1994.
18. Medicines Act, 1968; s92.
19. Medicines Act, 1968; s92 (5).
20. The Medicines (Advertising) Regulations, 1994; (SI 1994 No 1932) part IV.
21. Applebe GE, Wingfield J. *Pharmacy Law and Ethics*. 6th ed. The Pharmaceutical Press; p. 39.
22. Medicines Act 1968; s93 (7)(b).
23. R v Roussel Laboratories and another, 3 BMLR 128.
24. Anness v Grivell (1915) 3 KB 685; Barber v Cooperative Wholesale Society Ltd. (1983) Crim LR 476; Bastin v Davies (1950) 1 All ER 1095, 2KB 579, DC; Breed v British Drug Houses (1947) 2 All ER 613, DC; Goldup v John Manson Ltd. (1981) 3 All ER 257, (1982) QB 161, (1983) 3 WLR 833, DC; McDonald's Hamburgers v Windle (1987) 151 JP 333, DC; Shearer v Rowe (1985) 149 JP 698, DC.
25. PMCPA Constitution and Procedure; s1.1.
26. Ibid. s1.2.
27. 'Code of Practice for the Pharmaceutical Industry 1998'; Clause 1.1, Prescription Medicines Code of Practice Authority.
28. PMCPA Constitution and Procedure; s7.1.
29. R v British Pharmaceutical Industry Code of Practice Committee, Independent Law Report, 1 November 1990.
30. Associated Provincial Pictures Houses Ltd v Wednesbury Corporation [1948] 1 KB 223.
31. *Pharmaceutical Journal* 1998; **206**: 6.
32. Medicines Act 1968, s58.
33. The National Health Service (Charges for Drugs and Appliances) Amendment (No. 2) Regulations 2000: (SI 2000 No. 3189).
34. The Prescription Only Medicines (Human Use) Amendment Order 2003 (SI 2003 No 696).
35. www.medicines.mhra.gov.uk/inforesources/saleand supply/pgd.htm
36. Supplementary Prescribing by Nurses, Pharmacists, Chiropodists/ Podiatrists and Radiographers within the NHS in England: A guide to implementation. Department of Health, May 2005.
37. The Medicines for Human Use (Prescribing) (Miscellaneous Amendments) Order, 2005; (SI 2005 No. 1507).
38. Medicines Matters: A guide to mechanisms for the prescribing, supply and administration of medicines. Department of Health, National Practitioner Programme, July 2006.

Useful websites

Medicines and Healthcare Products Regulatory Agency: www.mhra.gov.uk
Royal Pharmaceutical Society of Great Britain: www.rpsgb.org.uk

UK Statutory Instruments: www.legislation.hmso.gov.uk/stat.htm

Electronic BNF: www.BNF.org

UK Acts of Parliament: www.legislation.hmso.gov.uk/acts.htm

UK Statutory Instruments: www.legislation.hmso.gov.uk/stat.htm

Scottish Statutory Instruments: www.scotland-legislation.hmso.gov.uk/
legislation/scotland/s-stat.htm

Scottish Acts of Parliament: www.scotland-legislation.hmso.gov.uk/
legislation/scotland/s-acts.htm

3 Evidence-based medicine

ANGELA TIMONEY

This chapter introduces the reader to the evidence-based philosophy of drug treatment, then considers how it can be used in practice, including current sources of information to inform clinical practice, the grading of evidence, and the integration of evidence into decision making.

Introduction

Medicines are used throughout the NHS to diagnose, cure or care for patients. It has been estimated that at any one time two thirds of the population are taking medicines. These may be prescribed products to treat chronic diseases or medicines purchased over the counter for short-term relief of minor ailments. As our understanding of medicines has increased, there has been an increasing awareness of the different clinical and cost effectiveness of the many drug choices available. When making a recommendation for a medicine, whether on prescription or for purchase, it is important to make that decision in a way that maximises the likely benefits and minimises the risks for the patient.

David Sackett, one of the founders of the evidence-based medicine philosophy, wrote that evidence-based medicine is: 'The conscientious, explicit and judicious use of current best evidence in making decisions about the care of individual patients.'[1]

Evidence-based medicine is therefore a way of bridging the gap between research and everyday practice and ensuring that clinical decisions are based on the best available scientific evidence. The definition is important because it recognises that information is used to inform decisions about an individual patient. It does not override the responsibility of the clinician for the patient and the need to recognise that often patients do not clearly or neatly fall into the categories described by the evidence. Judgments are required, but these judgements should be based on a thorough understanding of the evidence and the ability to assess how the evidence may be applied to the individual.

In the past it has been difficult for clinicians to collate and evaluate the evidence for practice. The medical literature, it has been suggested, is unwieldy, disorganised and biased, with many of the questions that arise in clinical practice unaddressed by well designed research.[2]

A systematic approach to gathering, collating, assessing and implementing evidence is therefore helpful for the individual and for the healthcare community as a whole. Systems are in place to collate this evidence, and this chapter describes these, including the types of medicines information available, the classification of evidence levels and the classification of grades of recommendations. A knowledge of and understanding of these systems and their levels enable the clinician to weigh the evidence when making decisions for patients.

Sources of clinical effectiveness information

There is a wealth of published literature available providing information on clinical efficacy and effectiveness of drug treatments. This has recently become more readily accessible through increasing use of the Internet. Literature can be classified in various ways; for example, as primary, secondary, or tertiary research or alternatively as 'white' or 'grey' literature. These terms are described in more detail below.

Primary research

Primary research describes clinical trials whereby the 'gold standard' is considered to be the *randomised controlled trial* (RCT). A controlled trial includes an intervention and a control group (also known as study arms). These two groups are required to be identical in every way except the treatment under investigation. Randomisation between the two arms ensures that each subject has an equal chance of being allocated to either group; therefore any factors likely to cause bias (known as confounding variables) should be equally distributed between groups.

RCTs may be:
- single-blinded (where the subjects are unaware of the arm they have been allocated to)
- double-blinded (where neither the subjects nor the investigators are aware of the arm the subject has been allocated to)
- open-label (where both subjects and investigators are aware of the arm the subject has been allocated to).

Blinding, theoretically, eliminates two major sources of bias: the investigator expecting an effect from a drug, or the patient expecting an effect, otherwise known as the 'placebo effect'. The placebo effect has variously been described as contributing approximately one third of the total observed effect.

Other types of clinical trials include:
- case-control studies – observational studies where characteristics of subjects with a disease are compared with a selected group of subjects without the disease
- cohort studies – observational studies of a group of subjects with a specific disease followed over time
- cross-sectional studies – surveys of the frequency of a disease or risk factor in a group of subjects at a single time point.

More information on study design is included in Chapter 6.

Secondary research

Secondary research is a term used to describe reviews of primary research, conducted to standard research principles, such as having a clearly articulated research question or hypothesis, a clearly described method, and objectively presented results from which conclusions can be logically drawn. The technique is referred to as systematic review.

Systematic reviews

Reviews can be anything from an individual specialist's overview of a subject, or a comprehensive literature review, to a systematic review. A systematic review indicates that the literature has been searched in a structured manner and has identified as far as possible all the relevant published papers that meet predefined quality standards; for example, only randomised clinical trials. These standards are described later in this chapter.

Whilst a systematic review can report its findings in a purely narrative or tabulated way, it is often associated with a statistical technique known as meta-analysis. This is an approach whereby data from a number of individual studies, judged to be sufficiently similar or homogeneous, is pooled numerically, generating one large virtual trial with greater statistical power than any of the studies alone. In this way, previously unknown effects may be identified, or confirmed with statistical confidence. The technique is particularly useful if the original trials involved few subjects and were unable to show a significant difference between intervention and control groups on their own.

There are various sources of systematic reviews, which are described below.

One of the first people to identify the hidden power of the data existing in the published literature was Archie Cochrane, and he inspired the establishment of the Cochrane Collaboration, represented in the UK by the UK *Cochrane Centre*. They publish excellent, highly regarded systematic reviews.

The Cochrane Library is a database of all the Cochrane Reviews that have been conducted. It is regarded as the most powerful source of evidence about the effects of healthcare anywhere in the world. It is published on a quarterly basis electronically on CD-ROM and on the Internet. Many countries, including all those in Great Britain, allow free access to The Cochrane Library through funded schemes. Reviews are not restricted solely to drug treatments but cover all types of health technologies enabling a comparison of the relative benefits of different types of treatment, such as medicines or surgery, for a given clinical problem. A topic for a review can be identified by any group of people who have identified a need for it; they then develop the review protocol, which has to be submitted to, and approved by the Cochrane Centre via one of the specialist editorial groups. Likewise the final review is sent out for peer review before final acceptance. One other important point is that all Cochrane reviews have to be regularly updated.

The *NHS Centre for Reviews and Dissemination* (CRD) at the University of York is also a useful source of information. It produces the *Database for Abstracts of Reviews of Effects* (DARE), which is a collection of structured abstracts of published, good quality systematic reviews available on the Internet. In addition it also provides two further databases, the NHS Economic Evaluation Database (NHS

EED) and the Health Technology Assessment (HTA) database.

One other interesting publication, available in paper and via the Internet, is *Bandolier* a short monthly journal containing systematic reviews and bullet points of evidence-based medicine, and of increasing interest to the GP population. As is the case with many electronic journals, the Bandolier Internet site contains more information than the paper journal and you can sign up to receive the contents of new editions by e-mail. The Internet version is free of charge but comes several months after the print version.

Other very useful reviews, which you may already be familiar with, include medicines information bulletins such as

- *MeReC Briefing*, produced by the National Prescribing Centre, Liverpool
- *Drug and Therapeutics Bulletin*, part of BMJ publications.

The latter two publications are available electronically on CD-ROM, giving an additional searching facility. In your local area, there may also be bulletins produced by Area Drug and Therapeutics Committees or Area Prescribing Committees. It is likely that these are supported by a thorough literature review.

Evidence-based guidelines

The Scottish Intercollegiate Guideline Network (SIGN) and the National Institute for Health and Clinical Excellence (NICE) are internationally recognised UK organisations producing guidelines for practice. The Canadian Agency for Drugs and Technologies in Health (CADTH), previously known as CCOHTA, also provides healthcare decision makers with important advice and evidence-based information about the effectiveness and efficiency of drugs and other health technologies. It is a highly regarded and useful information source.

These guidelines examine the evidence for a number of different interventions and collate this evidence to provide guidance for diagnosis and/or treatment of diseases or conditions.

In order for the evidence to be reviewed systematically, there must be agreement of the calibre of evidence and the weight given to different kinds of evidence. A common system for grading evidence and recommendations exists (*see* Tables 3.1 and 3.2 below).[3] This should be used to describe the level of evidence that supports any statement made in a guideline.

National Electronic Library for Health	http://www.nelh.nhs.uk
Bandolier	http://www.jr2.ox.ac.uk/bandolier
Cochrane Collaboration	http://hiru.mcmaster.ca/cochrane
Internet Grateful Med	http://igm.nlm.nih.gov
Joanna Briggs Institute	http://www.joannabriggs.edu.au
NHS Centre for Reviews and Dissemination	http://www.york.ac.uk/inst/crd
OMNI	http://www.omni.ac.uk
Pubmed	http://www4.ncbi.nlm.nih.gov/Pubmed
Scottish Medicines Consortium	http://www.scottishmedicines.org.uk
Scottish Intercollegiate Guideline Network	http://www.show.scot.nhs.uk/sign/
National Prescribing Centre	http://www.npc.co.uk
National Institute for Clinical Excellence	http://www.nice.org.uk
National Service Frameworks	http://www.nelh.nhs.uk/nsf

FIGURE 3.1 Useful websites

TABLE 3.1 Classification of evidence levels[3]

1++	High quality meta-analyses, systematic reviews of RCTs or RCTs with a very low risk of bias
1+	Well conducted meta-analyses, systematic reviews of RCTs, or RCTs with a low risk of bias
1-	Meta-analyses, systematic reviews of RCTs, or RCTs with a high risk of bias
2++	High quality systematic reviews of case-control or cohort studies
	High quality case-control or cohort studies with a very low risk of confounding, or bias and a moderate probability that the relationship is causal
2+	Well conducted case control or cohort studies with low risk of confounding, bias or chance and a moderate probability that the relationship is causal
2-	Case control or cohort studies with a high risk of confounding, bias or chance and a significant risk that the relationship is not causal.
3	Non-analytic studies, e.g. case reports, case series
4	Expert opinion

Thorough reviews of the literature are extremely time consuming, and are normally conducted by teams of people with duplicate reading of papers to maximise the reliability of the data reported. It is therefore sensible for an individual seeking information on which to make a clinical decision, to make good use of the sources of secondary research available. However, it is important to have confidence in the conclusions of reviews or guidelines that you choose to use. Even those produced by the bodies already mentioned earlier should be looked at critically, both for their methodological quality, the clinical significance of the conclusions, and the applicability of the conclusions to the population in question. Some tips to help you evaluate controlled trials are included later in this chapter. Even if you disagree with the conclusions of a review it should provide you with some useful references of the primary evidence.

TABLE 3.2 Classification of grades of recommendations[3]

A	At least one meta-analysis, systematic review or RCTs, or RCT rated as $1++$ and directly applicable to the target population; *or*
	A body of evidence consisting principally of studies rated as $1+$, directly applicable to the target population, and demonstrating consistency of overall results.
B	A body of evidence including studies rated as $2++$, directly applicable to the target population, and demonstrating overall consistency of results; *or*
	Extrapolated evidence from studies rated as $1++$ or $1+$
C	A body of evidence including studies rated as $2+$, directly applicable to the target population and demonstrating overall consistency of results; *or*
	Extrapolated evidence from studies rated as $2++$
D	Evidence level 3 or 4; *or*
	Extrapolated evidence from studies rated as $2+$

Note: The grade of recommendation relates to the strength of the evidence on which the recommendation is based. It does not reflect the clinical importance of the recommendation.

White and grey literature
In relation to literature, the terms white and grey describe publication status and, by inference, quality. White literature is published in peer reviewed journals, where at least two reviewers have critically appraised the submitted article and agree that it is of reasonable quality and should be published. Well known examples include:
- *The Lancet*
- *British Medical Journal (BMJ)*
- *New England Journal of Medicine (NEJM)*
- *Journal of the American Medical Association (JAMA).*

It should be noted, however, that some journal supplements may be sponsored or include articles, studies or abstracts not subject to the same peer review process as regular editions.

Grey literature includes other less rigorous publications such as:

- reports
- promotional material
- consensus based guidelines.

Although these may be very useful, they are often not peer reviewed, which questions the validity of their conclusions. Promotional material used to advertise medicines should be carefully studied. Beware of graphs where:

- axes do not start at zero
- inappropriate scales have been used
- data has been extrapolated (wasn't obtained directly from the study)
- there is an absence of error bars.

Check whether the references are from in-house trials or from peer reviewed journals. In-house trials are those that are conducted by the pharmaceutical company. In cases of new medicines, this may be the only data that is available to you, so interpret this with caution.

Literature searches

Despite the above cautions there will be times when dedicated self-conducted searches of the literature are necessary, seeking to identify both secondary and primary research of relevance. There is a definite skill to literature searching, and it has been said that even an experienced literature searcher may only identify half the relevant publications that are in the public domain. However, the route to the literature is becoming increasingly electronic, and thereby increasingly accessible. Many of the bulletins mentioned above are available on CD-ROM and incorporate a searching facility. Likewise, databases of systematic reviews or journals available on the Internet often incorporate a searching facility.

Forming a question

Before starting a search, formulate your question carefully and precisely, for example:

'What is the most effective treatment for condition X?'

or

'What is the evidence of efficacy relating to the new drug Y?'

As already explained, there is a huge volume of medical literature available, so you therefore need to make your question as narrow and as focused as possible. Considering the following types of questions should help.

■ Do I want to compare drug Y to existing therapy?
■ Do I want details of human studies only?
■ Do I want to exclude very short term studies?

Precise definition of the question will help you define your search strategy, using key words and headings to identify the most useful papers.

Electronic databases

There is a range of electronic databases available which include all publications from a declared list of journals. This is of importance if you need to source original clinical trials or reviews. The most relevant and well known in the field of medical literature is *Medline*, but others, for example, *CINAHL* (which has more of the nursing literature) and *International Pharmaceutical Abstracts* (IPA) may also include relevant papers. It is also important to do some hand searching of likely target journals, and to follow up references in the articles retrieved in the initial searches.

Internet sites such as PubMed can be used to search databases. PubMed is the US National Institutes of Health (NIH) digital archive of biomedical and life sciences journal literature. It has useful tutorials to instruct users on search terms, search strategies and so forth. This Internet route is easy to use and enables some filtering of trials. The databases usually provide abstracts of articles as well as titles. This limited information can allow some pre-screening of the papers identified by the original search (known as 'hits'). To interpret the study or review fully, you will need to obtain the complete article.

General Internet searches

The Internet contains a huge volume of information; it is possible to search the Internet by using various search engines, whereby each has its own instructions and 'tips' for searching. There is no censorship or control of information posted on the Internet. Most of the information will not have received any check on quality or veracity. There are, however, some useful health databases, such as Intute, which only contain information that adheres to certain quality criteria. Care should be taken before accepting information from Internet sites not maintained by a recognised body.

Sites identified using Intute will probably be more relevant and of more use to you. The disadvantages are that potentially useful resources may be overlooked and the database itself is relatively small.

Critical appraisal of the literature

As noted earlier in this chapter quality criteria must be applied to papers identified in the searches, before coming to a final conclusion. This is known as critical appraisal. It is important to establish validity prior to implementing any form of evidence. Whether evaluating a systematic review, a randomised controlled trial, an advertisement, or a guideline, the principles of critical appraisal are similar. The aim is to detect bias, that is to say, reasons why the conclusions drawn may not apply to the population as a whole. Various checklists exist to guide the reader through the critical evaluation process, such as those produced by Cochrane, or SIGN. An example is shown in Figure 3.2.

Key points to consider are summarised below.
- How was the study done?
- What are the results?
- How are the results presented?
- What are the conclusions?

How was the study done?

Firstly, the authors of the study should have stated the hypothesis or research question they wished to test; for example, is drug X significantly different from placebo? Ideally, all possible sources of bias should be eliminated. The perfect trial:
- is randomised
- is controlled
- is double blind (where both subjects and researchers are unaware which is the intervention group)
- measures a relevant clinical outcome as a primary endpoint. There should be a calculation of the 'power' of the study. This is the number of subjects that are required to enable the study to show a clinically significant difference between intervention and control

1. **Why – What is the question to be answered?**
1.1 Did the trial address a clearly focused issue?

2. **How was the trial carried out?**
2.1 Was the assignment of patients to treatments randomised?
2.2 Were all of the patients who entered the trial properly accounted for at its conclusion?
2.3 Were patients, health workers and study personnel 'blind' to treatment?
2.4 Were groups similar at the start of the trial?
2.5 Aside from the experimental intervention, were the groups treated equally?
2.6 Was the trial ethical?

3. **What are the results?**
3.1 How large was the treatment effect?
3.2 Was analysis carried out on an intention to treat basis?
3.3 What about the adverse effects?

4. **Will the research help locally? What is the relevance and implications?**
4.1 Can the results be applied to the local population?
4.2 Were all clinically important outcomes considered?
4.3 Are the benefits worth the harm and costs?

5. **Summary**

FIGURE 3.2   Critical appraisal checklist for a randomised controlled trial

groups and is usually expressed as a power between 80% and 90%. It is also worth looking at the population in which the trial was conducted, and whether this population is broadly similar to the one to which you will be applying the evidence.

Often trials measure surrogate (or proxy) markers rather than specific clinical end points. For example, when testing a drug for the treatment of gastrointestinal (GI) disease, a long-term clinical endpoint would be the number of serious GI events, e.g. GI bleeds, whereas a surrogate marker could be endoscopic changes. When testing an antiretroviral drug for the treatment of HIV, a long-term clinical endpoint would be death, whereas a surrogate marker could be white blood cell count or viral load.

Clinical outcomes, such as death, are far more important than changes in surrogate markers. Therefore to be valid there must be correlation between the surrogate endpoint and the clinical endpoint and the surrogate endpoint must fully capture the net effect of the treatment on the clinical endpoint.[4]

Caution is required when interpreting most, if not all, trials involving surrogate markers. For example, the benefits observed in long-term outcome trials of statins may be due to more than cholesterol lowering alone. Therefore a study that measures decrease in mortality is of higher quality than one that measures cholesterol alone. Higher quality evidence provides you with a higher quality recommendation for use.

Comparative trials may compare the efficacy of one drug against another (at comparable doses) or compare the drug to placebo. The former are of far more use than placebo controlled trials, but are only possible if there is already an established treatment. Advantages of placebo controlled trials are that it is easier to demonstrate superiority over placebo than over an established therapy, and smaller numbers of subjects are needed. Advantages of comparisons with standard treatments are that they are ethically preferable, and of more value if improved benefit can be demonstrated. Caution is required where comparative trials do not use comparable doses as this may show relatively better efficacy for one drug or relatively lower side effects.

What are the results?

Ideally, studies should be analysed by an 'intention to treat' method. This means that all subjects initially randomised are included in the final analysis and this takes account of subjects who withdrew and corresponds to the real life situation where patients fail to comply. Patients may withdraw from the study for a number of reasons, the most likely being due to adverse effects. Sometimes results are analysed by an 'on treatment' or 'per protocol' method, which means that only subjects who received, or remained on, treatment are analysed.

The primary endpoint should be the focus of the analysis. Be cautious where main findings are based on sub-group analyses not originally planned at the start of the study. This may be that the authors are 'data dredging', i.e. finding data to try to support a hypothesis.

How are the results presented?

This is where you are likely to come across some complex statistics.

For the purposes of this chapter, the terms are summarised and briefly explained below.

Significance tests

Significance tests are used to quantify the probability (p-value) that any observed difference between treatments could have occurred by chance. They don't *prove* that one treatment is better than another. Generally, a p-value below 0.05 indicates a true difference and is regarded as 'significant', whereas a p-value above 0.05 is regarded as non-significant. The 95% confidence interval (CI) is another way of presenting the same information. This is the range that includes the true value in 95% of cases.

Relative risk reduction

The clinical effectiveness of a treatment can be presented in a number of ways.

Study results are often presented in terms of relative risk reduction. This is the difference in event rate between the intervention and control group as a percentage of the control event rate. For example, in the 4S study,[5] which compared simvastatin to placebo in patients with angina or post MI, 8% of patients in the simvastatin group and 12% of patients in the placebo group died. Therefore the relative reduction in mortality achieved by simvastatin was 33%.

$$\text{i.e. } \frac{(\% \text{ died in placebo group}) - (\% \text{ died in simvastatin group})}{(\% \text{ died in placebo group})} \times 100$$

Absolute risk reduction

Absolute risk reduction is the percentage difference in event rate between the intervention and control groups. For example, in the 4S study (data given above) the absolute reduction in mortality achieved with simvastatin was 4%, i.e.

$$(\% \text{ died in placebo group}) - (\% \text{ died in simvastatin group})$$

It should be clear from these two examples that it is better to look at absolute not relative risk reduction. It is better to have a small reduction in a high risk than a large reduction in an extremely unlikely event.

Odds ratio (OR)

The odds ratio is the odds (ratio of probability) of an event happening in the intervention group divided by the odds of it occurring in the control group. If it equals one then the effects of the treatment are no different from those of the control. If the odds ratio is greater (or less) than one, then the effects of the treatment are more (or less) than those of the control. For example, using the 4S study once again, the mortality odds ratio achieved by simvastatin is 0.67.

$$\text{i.e. } \frac{(\% \text{ died in simvastatin group})}{(\% \text{ died in placebo group})}$$

Number needed to treat (NNT)

The expression 'number needed to treat' is a standardised way of describing the number of people you would need to treat to prevent one clinical event, such as death. For example, in the 4S study, when treating 100 people in each group, four fewer people in the test group died. For one extra person to have survived, 25 people would need to have been treated. The NNT is also arithmetically the reciprocal of the absolute risk reduction. The 4S study gives us a NNT of 25 to prevent one death by using simvastatin over a period of five years. It is a useful measure for putting trial results into perspective. We can use NNTs to gain a rough comparison of costs and benefits. For example, with an NNT of 25, prevention of one death with simvastatin at a dose of 10mg twice daily would cost 25 times the cost of 10mg twice daily for five years. Although it is possible to compare NNTs across similar interventions, you must remember that each NNT belongs to a particular trial of a particular duration.

Having calculated these different parameters of clinical effectiveness for the same study, you can see that the way that results are presented can influence how study results are perceived.

What are the conclusions of the study?

The discussion put forward by the authors should describe in detail any observed inconsistencies or shortcomings of the trial, and take these into account by considering the effects they might have had on the actual findings. Conclusions drawn should reflect what the study has actually shown, rather than what the authors would have liked it to demonstrate. You need to consider what the trial means clinically and whether the results can be applied to the general population. Sometimes study results show statistical but not clinical significance. For example, a blood pressure reduction of 3mmHg may be statistically significant but is meaningless clinically considering most blood pressure measurements are rounded down to the nearest 5mmHg.

Appraising a review

When appraising a review the principles are the same. In addition, you want to be sure that it is comprehensive by including all relevant trials. The criteria for including studies should be stated, and details should be provided if trials are omitted.

Publication bias is also a problem for reviewers. This is because studies showing that one drug has no advantage over another are often not accepted for publication, whilst studies that show more positive findings are published.

Similarly, when appraising guidelines, check that they cite the important trials. This may mean that you have to go back to the primary research sources via a Medline search, or check references cited in reviews conducted in the same area.

Current mechanisms to integrate evidence with decision making

After evidence has been gathered, collated, appraised and published there is still a requirement to try to ensure that evidence is then used. It has been shown that implementation is a separate discipline to that where the research evidence is gathered or that of guideline development where it is critically appraised. Professionals are influenced in their practice in numerous ways. For some the views of an opinion leader or an acknowledged expert will be influential, for others a critical incident in their practice will cause them to reflect, review and possibly change their approach. Grimshaw has concluded that there is an imperfect evidence base to support decisions about which guideline dissemination and implementation strategies are likely to be efficient under different circumstances.[6]

In the UK there are a number of bodies producing national guidance to enable good evidence to be available to contribute to decision making. These were referred to earlier and are described in more detail here, but you will need to consider carefully how to ensure this evidence is best used locally.

National Institute for Health and Clinical Excellence (NICE)

NICE was set up as a Special Health Authority in 1999. Its role is to provide patients, health professionals and the public with authoritative, robust and reliable guidance on current 'best practice'. It now provides guidance in three areas of health – public health, health technologies and clinical practice. In relation to medicines NICE produces multiple technology appraisals (MTA), which provide advice for clinical conditions, and single technology appraisal, which provide guidance usually regarding the use of a single medicine for a particular condition.

Scottish Medicines Consortium (SMC)

The SMC is a consortium of Area Drug and Therapeutics Committees (ADTCs) in Scotland. SMC comes under the umbrella of NHS Quality Improvement Scotland. The SMC remit states that it will 'provide advice to NHS Boards and the Area Drug and Therapeutics Committees (ADTCs) across Scotland about the status of all newly licensed medicines, all new formulations of existing medicines and new indications for existing products'. The SMC differs from many other advisory bodies on medicines in that it aims to get the information to prescribers, and other health care professionals, at or around the time of launch of the product. It is proposed by providing information at this time that prescribers will be supported in decision making when they first wish to use the product.

Scottish Intercollegiate Guidelines Network (SIGN)

The Scottish Intercollegiate guidelines Network (SIGN) aims to improve the quality of healthcare by reducing variation in practice and outcomes through the development and dissemination of national clinical guidelines containing recommendations for effective practice based on current evidence. The membership of SIGN comprises all medical specialties, nursing, pharmacy, dentistry, allied health professionals, patients, health service managers, social services and researchers. Over 90 SIGN guidelines are available and these can be downloaded free from the Internet. The website address is given at the end.[7]

National Service Frameworks (NSFs)

National Service Frameworks (NSFs) are another mechanism to integrate evidence with decision making and from there into practice.

NSFs are part of NHS policy in England and Wales and they set out to achieve the following:
- Set national standards and identify key interventions for a defined service or care group.
- Put in place strategies to support implementation.
- Establish ways to ensure progress within agreed timescales.
- Raise quality and decrease variations in service.

Conclusion

The production of information, and in particular health information, continues to grow apace. In order to harness this information with respect to the use of medicines it is important to understand and use a systematic approach to your practice. This begins by developing an understanding of evidence-based medicine. It can aid decision making but this must happen in the context of care for an individual. Next, with an understanding of the principles, practitioners should increase their knowledge and understanding of the types of evidence available and the advantages and disadvantages of each. With this background a systematic approach to searching for sources of information, for critically appraising it and developing it into guidance should be developed. Finally, the practitioner should enable this evidence to be used judiciously, for the benefit of patients. This chapter has attempted to take you through each of these stages, and to point you to the many resources now available to undertake much of this work. With the underpinning knowledge these resources can then be used and implemented with confidence.

References

1. Sackett DL, Richardson WS, Rosenberg W, Haynes RB. *Evidence-based Medicine. How to Practice and Teach EBM.* New York: Churchill Livingstone; 1998.
2. Getting evidence into practice. *BMJ* 1998; **317**: 6.
3. Harbour R, Miller J. A new system for grading recommendations in evidence-based guidelines. *BMJ* 2001; **323**: 334–6.
4. Fleming TR. Surrogate endpoints and FDA's accelerated approval process. *Health Affairs* 2005; **24**: 67–78.
5. Randomised trial of cholesterol lowering in 4444 patients with coronary heart disease: The Scandinavian Simvastatin Survival Study (4S). *Lancet* 1994; **344**: 1383–9.

6. Grimshaw J (2006). Effectiveness and efficiency of guideline dissemination and implementation strategies. *The Research Findings Register*. Summary number 1520. www.ReFeR.nhs.uk/ViewRecord.asp?ID=1520

7. Scottish Intercollegiate Guidelines Network. http://www.sign.ac.uk/

4 Clinical decision support systems

STUART McTAGGART

This chapter considers the nature of clinical decision support systems, describes some of the different types, and their value and application in clinical practice. There is consideration of some of the evaluation literature and the relevance of this implementation of decision support systems. Finally the chapter looks at the future for these systems and how they might develop.

Introduction

Computers are highly effective and efficient at storing and processing large amounts of information, consistently applying a set of rules to a situation or at performing routine and repetitive tasks without fatigue. Healthcare is a knowledge intensive industry; early on in the development of medical computing the potential was recognised for producing a computer that could match or even surpass the abilities of a human clinician. The focus has changed somewhat to developing systems that aid rather than replace the clinician and with the increasing availability in electronic format of information about medical knowledge and the individual patient, the importance of such aids is only likely to increase.

This chapter will consider what clinical decision support systems (CDSS) are, why they are needed and the principles upon which they operate. It will look at systems in clinical use, with a particular emphasis on those systems involving prescribing of drugs and at the benefits or otherwise that such systems have been shown to bring, including the effect on clinician-patient interaction. Finally, there will be a short discussion of how CDSS might develop in the future and the factors likely to influence this.

What are clinical decision support systems?

Clinical decision support systems have been broadly defined as any computer program that helps health professionals to make clinical decisions. However, this definition is quite wide-ranging and could include electronic guidelines or electronic texts such as the Electronic British National Formulary (eBNF) and does not encompass the concept that CDSS should be used in the care of individual patients. A better definition might be computer software employing a knowledge base designed for use by a clinician involved in patient care, as a direct aid to decision making.

CDSS differ from guidelines, protocols or care management pathways in that they require the input of patient specific data and result in an output that is relevant to that particular patient. However, they draw on the evidence-based literature described in Chapter 3.

How CDSS work

CDSS have typically been developed to address specific functions such as to aid prescribing, manage specific disease areas or to aid the interpretation of laboratory tests. Such systems are sometimes referred to as expert systems. The system will include a knowledge base and a method of applying that knowledge and, because CDSS provide information relevant to the care of an individual patient, the system must have some means of gathering information about that patient. This could be through the use of on-screen prompts to the clinician or by directly reading information from the electronic health record (EHR). Several features of CDSS have been identified.[1] They should:

■ provide a solution at the same level of performance as a human expert
■ use symbolic and heuristic (rule of thumb) reasoning rather than numeric and algorithmic procedures
■ store knowledge separately from inference procedures
■ provide explanations of their reasoning.

Currently three types of expert system have been developed: rule based systems, probabilistic systems, and cognitive models.[1] These are described below:

1. *Rule-based systems* present information in context and in response to a series of problem-led prompts that may guide choice of drug, provide reminders, or suggest diagnostic strategies. Rules may be based on clinical or demographic characteristics, combinations of features, or results of previous steps. They may be more an aid to communication than to the logical application of knowledge. Such systems promote learning and involvement in the diagnostic process and hence are likely to be used more than systems that hide their rules.

   PRODIGY (prescribing rationally with decision support in general practice study) is an example of a rules-based CDSS in clinical use.[2] PRODIGY provides decision support to general practitioners within the consultation regarding appropriate drug choices based on diagnosis. The system also supports nurse prescribing and includes information leaflets for patients about the condition and its treatment.

   Simple rule-based systems are likely to be supplanted in the future by probabilistic systems, which are described next.

2. *Probabilistic systems* model patient data against epidemiological data to predict future events, either for prognostic or diagnostic purposes. Such systems, however, are limited by both the availability of data and the complexity of possible outcomes. Many specialties lack prognostic information while few specialties have access to true baseline data. Probabilistic systems separate knowledge from inference and can be readily updated. For example rather than considering hypertension, smoking, or hyperlipidaemia in isolation, the risk of a cardiovascular event or mortality can be calculated for an individual patient from Framingham data. Such risk charts are published in the *British National Formulary* (BNF) and are available on the *BNF* website.[3]

3. *Simulation models* consider a system or reality in terms of states, with a change of state referred to as an event (e.g. a 'healthy' person contracts a disease). A patient's life cycle can be divided into a series of events and their passage determined by estimated probabilities. Such simulations can operate at an individual patient level. This allows modelling of the outcome for an individual patient following different diagnoses or interventions.

Like probabilistic models, simulation models are hampered by our imperfect knowledge. However, simulation models offer the potential to develop CDSS that learn from events and can develop and test new hypotheses about treatment options and so improve the effectiveness of probabilistic model based systems. Medical care is an information rich process and increasing amounts of this information are recorded and stored electronically in standardised ways. Computers are extremely effective at processing and sifting through large amounts of data and so could be used to discover new associations between interventions and outcomes, particularly in terms of the effectiveness of drug treatments in actual clinical use as opposed to the controlled circumstances of a clinical trial.

Why CDSS are needed

The provision of healthcare is a knowledge-intensive industry yet it is often left up to individual practitioners to ensure that they are aware of relevant advances in medicine and the latest developments in evidence-based medicine and guidelines for best practice. CDSS help clinicians apply what science has learned and so frees the professional from the unrealistic expectation that the unaided human mind can stay current with the approximately 20,000 new articles that appear in the biomedical literature every year.

Much of modern healthcare takes place in the primary care setting and it is the GP who most often sees the initial presentation of a disease, when there is the greatest level of uncertainty about the diagnosis. GPs are also responsible for the majority of the management of chronic conditions. Whilst individual GPs may specialise in certain disease areas they still need to maintain an up to date knowledge over most areas of medicine and drug therapy and so can gain benefit from CDSS. Within the acute healthcare setting, much of the hands-on medical care is carried out by junior doctors. Such doctors have limited experience and may have gaps in their knowledge. Specialist consultants have in-depth knowledge about specific diseases and their treatments but are often distant from the patient, particularly at initial presentation. Clinical decision support tools have the potential to be the expert in the surgery or A&E department, particularly for the more unusual or ambiguous cases.

Adverse drug events or errors involving drugs are known to be a significant cause of morbidity and mortality and in many cases are preventable.[4] Such events can include drug-drug interactions, drug disease interaction/contraindication, and drug dosage errors. Whilst some of these could not have been predicted, many may be the result of imperfect knowledge or poor application of knowledge by the clinician, and could therefore be considered avoidable. A meta-analysis reported an incidence of 6.7% for serious adverse events, a description that excludes errors. It has been suggested that between 28% and 56% of adverse drug events are preventable.[5]

In summary, CDSS may support the clinical process in the following ways:[1,6]

- by giving ready access to appropriate knowledge and protocols based on patient specific prompts
- by providing a rational aid to diagnosis or probable outcome based on patient specific data
- by involving patients explicitly in the decision making process.

Additional benefits may include:
- improved patient safety through interaction, contraindication and dose checking for drugs
- release of staff and increased accuracy through the automation of repetitive or tedious tasks
- less variation in standards of care and improved compliance with best practice leading to improved patient outcomes
- reduced costs and improved efficiency through the more rational use of drugs and discouraging inappropriate ordering of tests.

Application of CDSS

Depending on the design of the system and the circumstances of use CDSS can be described as active or passive. Active systems are always on and operate in the background, producing an alert of some sort when they detect a potential problem. An example of such a system might be an interaction checking system that monitors the prescribing of drugs and produces an alert when a potential interaction is detected.[7] The Multilex drug knowledge-base produced by First Databank Europe is widely used within clinical systems in the UK and is most often implemented as an active system.[8] Passive systems, on the other hand, need to be invoked by the user. A tool that aids diagnosis might be such a system as it will not always be required but will be used only in cases of uncertainty. There are many areas to which CDSS can be applied.[7]

Alerts and reminders

A system might scan test or laboratory results and by way of on-screen prompts or e-mail alert the clinician to important changes; for example, hypokalaemia or a falling potassium level in a patient receiving digoxin. A reminder system might alert a clinician that a patient is eligible for and has not yet received their winter flu vaccination.

Diagnostic aids

When a patient's case is complex, rare or the person making the diagnosis is simply inexperienced an expert system can be helpful. Likely diagnoses are formulated based on patient data and the system's understanding of disease stored in its knowledge base.

Therapy critiquing and planning

Critiquing systems can look for inconsistencies, errors or omissions in a patient's treatment but they do not offer actual guidance about how the patient should be treated. For example, on ordering a blood transfusion the system might inform the clinician that the patient's haemaglobin level is above the transfusion threshold and prompt for an indication such as active bleeding. Planning systems have more knowledge of treatment protocols and so can help to formulate an appropriate care plan using patient specific data from the EHR and accepted treatment guidelines.

Prescribing decision support systems (PDSS)

Prescribing of drugs is a common clinical task and unsurprisingly it is probably the area that has seen the most widespread use of decision support software. PDSS can help in the prescribing process by checking for drug-drug interactions, dosage errors and, where connected to the EHR, for other contraindications such as drug allergy checking. Such systems are usually well received because they support a routine task and as well as improving the clinical quality of that task they also offer additional benefits such as improved legibility of prescriptions, a complete and easily retrievable prescribing record and electronic transmission of the prescription.

Evaluation of CDSS

A number of studies have investigated the impact of CDSS but these are often specific in their focus, such as the impact on consultation times or the effect on adherence to treatment guidelines, and few studies assessed the impact of CDSS on patient outcomes. The general evidence for CDSS being of benefit is there, but if it forms part of the clinical intervention then surely it must be subject to the same level of evidence-based scrutiny as any other intervention.

A review of the use of computers in primary care identified 90 prospective studies that investigated the effect of computers on the consultation process, on general practitioners' task performance, on patient outcomes or on doctors' or patients' attitudes to computerisation.[9] The review was not confined to CDSS but many of the studies included CDSS functions. In addition, several studies evaluated the impact of the computer on the content and dynamics of the consultation and this provided insights that might be applicable to CDSS. The use of computers in the consultation increased the length of the consultation by an average of 90 seconds but this decreased over time, returning to baseline on average after 30 days. There was an increase in the amount of practitioner-centred speech and an increase in the number of medical topics raised. This was often at the expense of patient orientated activity and in one study patients appeared to synchronise their speech with perceived pauses in practitioner keyboard activity.

Several studies investigated the impact of reminders and prompts for preventative tasks such as blood pressure measurements. Practitioner performance increased by up to 47% and the greatest improvements were seen when practitioners were prompted as part of the consultation. Disease management was improved with the use of electronic protocols with improvements of up to 69% in the management of diabetes and up to 53% in managing hypertension. However, these improvements came at the cost of a longer consultation, increased by 10 minutes for diabetes and by one third for hypertension. The use of computers increased the use of generic drugs, reduced prescribing costs and freed up practitioner and receptionist time. Computer use for ordering tests reduced the number of tests ordered as well as costs.

Few studies have looked at the effect on actual patient outcomes, and conclusions are mixed. The use of computers in the management of hypertension resulted in significantly more patients with reduced diastolic pressure whereas whilst one study found an improvement in anticoagulant management, another did not. There was no evidence that the use of computers led to an increase in service use in terms of visits to primary care or referrals to secondary care and one study detected a shift whereby patients in computerised practices were managed more in the community. An evaluation of decision support for lipid management found a 55% reduction in the number of expected referrals.

CDSS in clinical use

The basis for CDSS, that healthcare workers require assistance because they are either prone to error or their efficiency could be improved and that assistance could be provided by computer systems that mimic or emulate at least part of the process considered to belong to the human intellect, seems to be a reasonable assumption. Indeed the body of evidence supports the hypothesis that CDSS are beneficial to the healthcare process and these benefits can be divided into the following three broad areas.[7]

- Improved patient safety through reduced medication errors and adverse events and improved medication and test ordering.
- Improved quality of care by increased application of clinical pathways and guidelines, facilitating the use of up to date clinical evidence and improving clinical documentation.
- Improved efficiency in healthcare delivery by reducing costs through faster order processing, decreased test duplication, decreased adverse events and changed patterns of prescribing favouring cheaper but equally effective generic drugs.

Why then are CDSS not in more widespread clinical use? It has been suggested that this may be the result of clinicians being unaware of the benefits that such systems can bring, that the available systems do not meet the needs of clinicians or, most contentiously, the technophobia or computer illiteracy of healthcare workers.[10] Many areas of healthcare are innovative and use leading edge technologies that have been embraced by clinicians and so the last suggestion would seem unlikely. As has been discussed previously, there is an increasing body of evidence that CDSS bring a number of benefits and much of this has been published in mainstream medical journals. Finally, where it has been assessed, practitioners and patients have generally expressed satisfaction with the use of CDSS. Perhaps the answer to this puzzle lies in access to computers and scalability?

Two papers by Benson[11,12] highlight the main reasons why

computers have been universally adopted in primary care but less so in secondary care.

- Because of the differences in how primary care and secondary care are funded there has been a business need for primary care clinicians to use computers to record information.
- Primary care clinicians often work from a fixed location (which allows installation and access to a computer) whereas secondary care clinicians may provide care from a variety of settings (patient bedside, outpatient clinics, etc.).
- Primary care is in some ways more predictable and limited in the range of tasks that are covered.
- Primary care establishments are small and so introducing a computer system is relatively straightforward and most primary care facilities are quite similar in nature.
- Hospitals are far more complex and the set-up may vary not only between hospitals but between specialties within the same site.

More recently, the new GMS contract and the Quality and Outcomes Framework necessitates the availability of electronic clinical information in a number of disease areas and will undoubtedly further improve the quantity and quality of information recorded electronically and encourage 'paperless' practice. The computer and electronic health record are increasingly a natural part of the consultation.

The widespread availability of computers, the increasing amount of electronic clinical information available and the use of these within the primary care consultation give a sound environment for introducing CDSS. Prescribing is one of the most frequent tasks undertaken in general practice and electronic prescribing has been shown to improve the clarity of prescriptions, reduce errors and release staff time. If prescription information is being stored electronically, it is a relatively small step to introduce drug-drug interaction checking and this has been a feature of GP and pharmacy systems for many years. As the volume of electronically recorded clinical information increased then it also became possible to introduce new features such as allergy and contraindication checking.

In comparison with secondary care, primary care facilities such as a GP practice are very small and perform a limited range of functions. The amount of data and the uses to which it must be put are fewer and it is the norm to have a single integrated system. Designing systems to store and display this information becomes less complex and most

GP systems have an active user community with similar needs who are often very willing to be involved in development.

By contrast, computer use within UK hospitals is much more limited and often confined to specific tasks or functions and to individual units. Very few clinicians consult an electronic patient record and only a minority of drug orders are generated electronically.

How might CDSS develop?

Until now CDSS has been limited by the lack of standards in how clinical information is recorded and the terminologies and codes used to record that information. In the UK there has been no standard way of describing medicines and no standardised coding system so that while a human might recognise aspirin 75mg enteric-coated tablets and aspirin gastro-resistant tablets 75mg* as being the same thing, a computer would have considerable difficulty in so doing. Furthermore, rather than work with these cumbersome pieces of text, a computer will work with codes to represent these concepts. However, without a standardised coding system, even if the text is the same, the code used to represent it within one computer system will be different from that used in another. In addition, it is inefficient to hold knowledge about medicines against each individual preparation and so information may be held against some other attribute. For example, medicines containing aspirin have a common set of properties or all enteric-coated preparations should be swallowed whole and the patient counselled on this point. This adds relationships and structure to the data and so the knowledge bases used for CDSS start to become inextricably linked. For example, an interaction-checking program that stores information about the actual drug substance will only operate if it knows that 'Caprin', for example, is one of many different proprietary brands of aspirin. Most existing prescribing decision support systems have been designed to work with a specific drug dictionary and will normally have been developed by the vendor of that dictionary. Furthermore, there may have been some customisation or other development to allow them to be incorporated into a clinical application.

---

* Enteric-coated tablets have a special coating preventing the tablet from dissolving in the gastric acid of the stomach. Gastro-resistant is a more modern and broader term that can describe any formulation method to prevent dissolution in the stomach.

A number of products and technologies that will become more widely used over the next few years may change this, making it much more possible to 'mix and match' systems and to make the relevant information more available in the clinical setting.

Within England, the National Programme for Information Technology (NPfIT), now known as Connecting for Health (CfH)[13] brings increased standardisation in the way that patient specific information is expressed and stored and encourages the collection of clinical information. This provides a strong base from which to develop CDSS and indeed NPfIT has awarded a contract to First Databank Europe for it to provide its CDSS product.[14]

Electronic drug dictionaries

The development of the NHS Dictionary of Medicines and Devices (dm+d)[15] creates a unique and publicly available identifier for medicines and devices and so facilitates information exchange between systems that use the dm+d. The dm+d is set to become a national standard within the UK and will be at the heart of any systems that include a prescribing function or need to use information about the medicines that a patient is receiving. However, from the data architecture of the dm+d[15] and the underlying SNOMED-CT terminology[16] a system that receives a dm+d identifier for a medicine can *know* much more than simply what medicine that patient is receiving. For example, a system receiving a message that a patient has been prescribed Prozac 20mg capsules can also know that this is fluoxetine 20mg capsules and that fluoxetine is a serotonin re-uptake inhibitor and that this is a type of antidepressant.

Because each record and attribute within the dm+d has a unique and publicly available identifier, third parties can build decision support tools that link into this information about medicines without the need to build and maintain a drug dictionary of their own. As building and maintaining a drug dictionary represents a significant effort and cost, the removal of the need to do this could make it economical to develop specialist databases that link in with the dm+d. Examples could be CDSS for drug use in pregnancy and breast-feeding or drug use in renal disease.

The ever improving speed and reliability of communications networks means that acceptable levels of performance can occur even when most of an application is on a remote server. For example, using dm+d identifiers, the prescribing application could send a list of medicines that the patient is receiving to a specialist interactions checking application. This would perform checks for interactions and would return to the prescribing system a message that identified and gave details of any potential interactions. The clinician could then act on that information as appropriate. This type of system is known as web services and relies on published interfaces so that any application using the service can be designed to send the appropriate information needed by the web service, and to know what information to expect in return and in what format. The application sending information can be customised in how it responds to the information that it receives from the web service. Multiple web services could be used to cover different aspects of decision support, for example interaction checking, contraindication checking, dosage advice, etc. Making use of this type of service presents no risk to patient confidentiality as no patient identifiable information need be sent to the web service. In the interaction checking example, all that is needed is the name of the medicine about to be prescribed together with a list of the other medicines that the patient is receiving but nothing else about the patient.

Use of hand-held devices

While much of primary care is conducted at the clinician's desk a significant amount of interactions occur at remote locations such as the patient's home and by a variety of clinicians. Hand-held mobile devices and the use of Internet technologies will allow these clinicians to access patient information and CDSS at the point of patient care. By using secure communications technologies the hand-held device can access data at the surgery and make use of CDSS on the main system. In addition, any interventions made during the home visit can be recorded. By using secure Internet technologies and a web-browser, no patient data is permanently stored on the hand-held device and so there is no risk to patient confidentiality if the device is lost or stolen. These types of technology are also likely to be widely used in the hospital setting where care may take place in a wide variety of locations and where there can be a much greater need to share information across a team, so that storage of patient data on a central server or other integrated system allows remote access by multiple authorised users. Again, because no patient information is permanently stored on the hand-held device then there is no risk to patient confidentiality. Indeed, it could be argued that such a system is more secure than traditional paper case-notes that may be left unattended in wards and clinics.

The hospital setting

The use of CDSS will increase and the fastest growth is likely to be in the hospital setting (*see also* Chapter 10). Hospitals are increasingly employing electronic prescribing and this will contribute to the core patient record as part of NPfIT/CfH. CDSS is likely to be introduced at the same time as or shortly after electronic prescribing systems. NPfIT/CfH seeks to enforce standards and this would seem to extend to the provision of CDSS. However, it is likely that while this approach will simplify the introduction of CDSS across the NHS, user demands will become more sophisticated and specialist solutions will be developed based upon common standards and core systems.

Conclusion

CDSS has generally been shown to offer benefits to clinicians and patients but gaps have been identified. While initially the focus was on systems that aided complex diagnoses, the emphasis has now changed to systems that aid repetitive tasks such as prescribing and reducing risks to patients by, for example, interaction or dose checking. Systems are also being developed that incorporate the latest evidence-based guidelines and aid the clinician in selecting the best medicine for a particular patient.

Electronic prescribing with varying degrees of decision support is the norm in primary care within the UK but is still the exception in secondary care. The development of the dm+d and the NPfIT/CfH in England will see electronic prescribing develop further in secondary care and NPfIT/CfH will encourage the recording of clinical information to national standards. This improved repository of patient specific electronic clinical information will enable CDSS to be developed further. In addition, the huge data repository of diseases and prescribing that NPfIT/CfH will create will offer a fantastic opportunity for the development of CDSS systems that interrogate this information to assess the impact of interventions on patient outcomes and to identify the optimal interventions. This information will inform the knowledge bases used by the CDSS utilised by clinicians in the care of individual patients.

References

1. Delaney BC, Fitzmaurice DA, Riaz A *et al.* Can computerised decision support systems deliver improved quality in primary care? *BMJ* 1999; **319**: 1261–3.
2. Prodigy Knowledge. www.prodigy.nhs.uk
3. Mehta DK (Ed). *British National Formulary 51.* London: BMJ Publishing Group Limited & London: RPS Publications; 2006. www.bnf.org
4. Bates DW. Using information technology to reduce rates of medication errors in hospitals. *BMJ* 2000; **320**: 788–91.
5. Bates DW, Cullen DJ, Laird N *et al.* Incidence of adverse drug events and potential adverse drug events: implications for prevention. *JAMA* 1995; **274**: 29–34.
6. Payne TH. Clinical decision support systems. *Chest* 2000; **118**(Suppl.): 47S–52S.
7. Coiera E. Clinical decision support systems. In: Coiera E, editor. *Guide to Health Informatics: second edition.* Hodder Arnold; 2003.
8. First Databank Europe Ltd. www.firstdatabank.co.uk
9. Mitchell E, Sullivan F. A descriptive feast but an evaluative famine: systematic review of published articles on primary care computing during 1980–97. *BMJ* 2001; **322**: 279–82.
10. Coiera E. Question the assumptions. In: Barahono P, Christensen JP, editors. *Knowledge and Decisions in Health Telematics – the next decade.* Amsterdam: IOS Press; 1994.
11. Benson T. Why general practitioners use computers and hospital doctors do not – part 2: scalability. *BMJ* 2002; **325**: 1090–3.
12. Benson T. Why general practitioners use computers and hospital doctors do not – part 1: incentives. *BMJ* 2002; **325**: 1086–9.
13. Connecting for Health. www.connectingforhealth.nhs.uk
14. FDBE awarded contract by BT to support NHS Care Records Service; 2003 (News Article). www.firstdatabank.co.uk
15. NHS Dictionary of Medicines and Devices. www.dmd.nhs.uk
16. SNOMED Clinical Terms. www.snomedct.org

5 Online information systems

NICOLA GRAY AND ALISON BLENKINSOPP

This chapter informs a greater understanding of the needs of different lay and professional users of online medicines information, and describes the main types of medicines information available online and key web resources. It gives criteria for use in assessing quality of online medicines information, cites useful online medicines information sources for the public, and considers the current limitations of online medicines information, including the implications of health literacy.

Introduction

The Internet has the potential to facilitate public access to medicines information hitherto only available through specialist publications and/or from professionals. The implications of this are wide ranging, and most particularly affect the power dynamic of the professional-client relationship. This is reflected in other sociocultural changes and healthcare strategies. However, there are also other perspectives including the burgeoning increase in online information, meeting the needs of the heterogeneous group of people who use it, and its accessibility and quality. These perspectives provide the focus for further discussion in this chapter.

Who are the information users?

We have identified at least four main users of online medicines information:

- medicines consumer/patient
- practitioner/adviser
- prescriber
- policy maker/resource allocator.

Within each audience, there are levels of engagement that may also affect online proficiency. For example, an individual who is newly diagnosed with a long-term condition involving regular medication will have different needs and expertise than an 'expert patient' who has negotiated a stable self-management package with their care providers. There is some evidence to suggest that many people search for online health information on behalf of a member of their family or social circle. The most experienced Internet users in a household may be the younger members, but their relative lack of experience of illness and medicines may pose a challenge because of limited ability to evaluate what they find.

The prevalence of consumer use of the Internet for health information has been estimated as 21% in Australia,[1] and 27–31% in the US.[2] One study found that although a group of health information seekers rated the Internet positively as a source, many were unable to locate satisfactory information for a specific query.[3] The authors concluded that a key reason for positive attitudes despite mixed results was the consumers' unmet need through traditional channels, such as talking to health professionals.

A recent large public survey in the UK found that the Internet was a preferred source of health information about self-care for 12% and that a further 6% wanted to use it more in the future.[4] However, the survey also concluded that 'those least likely to have access to the Internet (the elderly and most socio-economically deprived) also tend to be the "poorest" in terms of using self-care information'.

Health professionals' use of the Internet varies considerably. It seems to be generally acknowledged that work-based use of the Internet has been adopted more slowly by health professionals than by some other occupational groups although evidence to support this assertion is scanty. Health professionals may access medicines information via the Internet for a number of reasons including decision support (*see also* Chapter 4), to obtain information for patients and for continuing professional development. A particular challenge is the need for rapid access during standard consultations and it has been suggested that in an 'average' GP consultation of 7–8 minutes, unless information can be obtained within 30 seconds, it is unlikely to be sought.

A survey of UK general practitioners published in 1998 found that 17% reported having access to the Internet in their surgery.[5] Canadian nurses' use of the Internet to 'look up nursing information' in a 1998 survey was found to be 16.5% at home and 5.1% at work.[6] A national US study of physicians found that 61% used the Internet in their practice,[7] mostly to find articles/guidelines, or to contact colleagues by e-mail. The authors commented that few respondents to their survey used the Internet to e-mail patients, or to access their laboratory test results.

We found no published research relating to the use of medicines information by policymakers or resource allocators. Whilst the use of the Internet for many consumers and clinicians is to find thera-peutic options and information for individuals, its potential to supply population-based medicine information appears to be relatively undeveloped. Certainly, policymakers have rapid access to pre-scribing guidelines and frameworks, but few other resources exist. In England, for example, prescribing advisers in NHS primary care organisations can access prescribing data for their locality online through ePACT (Electronic Prescribing Analysis and Costs) (*see also* Chapter 7). An international open-access journal established in 1993, 'Cost Effectiveness and Resource Allocation',[8] is aimed at policymakers and resource allocators. In addition to articles about different health conditions and service costs, medicines are also reviewed. In the light of the lack of peer-reviewed material aimed at this audience, but with many examples of good practice and institutional guidelines freely available, the policymaker needs also to review the relevance and credibility of each search that they undertake. The National Health Service's National Electronic Library for Health (NeLH)[9] website brought together a number of evidence sources including the Cochrane Library and the National Institute for Clinical Excellence. The NeLH has now been replaced by the National Library for Health (NLH).

The motivator: why is information needed?

Understanding the motivation for different medicines information users to go online is a key to improving that information and assessing the success of the search. The audiences we identified earlier in this chapter are not mutually exclusive, but their ability to locate and use

TABLE 5.1 Medicines information needs and audiences

PURPOSE		MEDICINES USERS / PATIENTS	PRESCRIBERS	PRACTITIONERS / ADVISERS	POLICYMAKERS/ RESOURCE ALLOCATORS	USEFUL SITES
Is a medicine needed?		'I have a problem and want to know if there is a treatment I can take for it.'	'I want to know what the latest evidence is for the use of medicines for this condition.'	'The patient has asked me whether a medicine is the only option in this condition.'	'Could self-care be a first-line recommendation here?'	eBNF NICE BestTreatments DI Zone
Choosing the medicine		'What are the alternatives to my treatment? Are they allowed on the NHS?' 'What's new for my condition? Is it allowed on the NHS?'	'What is the best treatment for my patient's condition?' 'Is there a clinical guideline for this condition?'	'The patient has asked me about a medicine prescribed from the hospital. It's not one I'm familiar with.'	'Should this new medicine be added to the formulary?'	NICE BestTreatments NLH guideline finder
Living with the medicine	Efficacy	'I've been taking a regular medicine for several months – how do I know if it's working?'	'My patient is due for a medication review. What monitoring tests do I need to do? What are successful treatment outcomes?'	'How is this patient coping with this medicine? Are they taking it?'	'Is there a NICE guideline for this condition?'	Emc BestTreatments NICE DiPEx
	Side effects	'I've experienced a side effect with my medicine. Have other people had the same problem. Should I change the medicine?'	'A medicine that I prescribe has been changed / discontinued / withdrawn for safety reasons. What are the alternatives?'	'A patient has asked me how likely they are to get a particular side effect.'	'Why has this medicine been withdrawn and do I need to do anything about it?'	DiPEx MHRA NPC

PURPOSE	MEDICINES USERS / PATIENTS	PRESCRIBERS	PRACTITIONERS / ADVISERS	POLICYMAKERS/ RESOURCE ALLOCATORS	USEFUL SITES
Availability	'I want to know if I can get the medicine that I want online.'	'Can my patient buy this OTC next time?'	'Is this medicine from the hospital available on FP10?'	'If this medicine is not available, are there any alternatives?'	netDoctor
Patterns of use		'How does my prescribing compare to others in my PCT?'		'How can we make the best use of our budget next year?'	

relevant and credible medicines information will be dependent upon factors such as existing Internet skills, awareness of potentially useful sites and health literacy.

In an Australian study of consumer use of the Internet for health information conducted in 2000 the commonest types of information sought were on the cause or nature of a disease or health condition (60%), then management or treatment (45%), complementary therapy alternatives (18%), over the counter medicines (10%) and support groups (9%).[1]

Table 5.1 illustrates the types of information that Internet users might seek and shows the different perspectives from which the same information might be accessed.

Perceived risk is an important motivator for consumers to access online medicines information, and there are issues relating to the way that they might cope with conflicting information. For example, a consumer might be more willing to purchase complementary medicines or non-prescription medicines online than a prescription medicine because the latter is perceived as inherently more potent and potentially more dangerous. A patient who is concerned about the adverse effects of their prescription therapy may visit several sites to corroborate evidence from the experiences of others in order to make their case with their prescriber or support their own decision about whether to continue treatment.

Perceptions of risk in relation to medicines are complex to unravel, and are likely to be dependent upon several factors including the individual's previous experience of a medicine, the seriousness of the condition, and the choice of treatments available for that condition. Even the concept of 'risk' is subject to interpretation: the consumer may be more concerned about a lack of efficacy, or risk of disappointment, than the probability of adverse effects.[10] It is likely that consumers do acknowledge a greater risk in the context of prescription medicines, notably recognition of the possibility of side effects. At the other extreme, however, a perception of all complementary/alternative medicines as 'safe' and 'natural' may persist.

The message – content of online sources

We have identified three broad categories of medicines-related infor-mation: clinical, administrative (e.g. over the counter availability) and retail (e.g. purchasing of medicines from online pharmacies). Research conducted pre-Internet on consumer judgements on credibility of information sources on non-prescription medicines found three key attributes: empathy, expertise and trustworthiness.[11] In our view this framework is highly relevant to consideration of the use of Internet-based medicines information and it will be used throughout the rest of this chapter.

Clinical

The UK has a National Health Service with a strong identity for consumers and professionals alike, and there are several NHS sites that provide information about medicines which can be accessed by lay as well as by health professional users. These may be dedicated medicine resources, such as UK Medicines Information, or sections within wider health reference sources, such as the treatment sections in NHS Direct Online's Health Encyclopaedia[12] or treatment guidelines within the National Institute for Health and Clinical Excellence (NICE) website.[13] It is notable that the National Electronic Library for Health (NeLH)[9] developed a specialist National Electronic Library for Medicines (NeLM),[14] which formerly existed as DrugInfoZone, and is now found on the National Library for Health website. Trustworthiness and expertise are likely to be high for both consumer and professional audiences. Empathy is likely to be higher for sites where consumers are the target audience than for some sites where content makes assumptions about existing knowledge.

Administrative

The development of online appointment booking systems is under way in the NHS and patients will in future be able to order repeat prescriptions online. In primary care some medical practices already operate an e-mail ordering system for repeat prescriptions. The NHS plans to provide 'My Health Space' for patients to record key information. Access will be controlled by the patient, and health professionals will need consent to view the information. Potentially 'My Health Space' offers the opportunity for access to patient-specific information such as on allergies to medicines, and about previous adverse effects.

Retail

Much information about medicines on the Internet is linked to advertising for certain products and ultimate online purchase. It is possible to obtain many medicines legally and ethically through online means, including personal importation of medicines from abroad. UK online pharmacies have developed mechanisms for dispensing NHS and private prescriptions under the current legal and regulatory framework. This is likely to develop further, following the trials for electronic transfer of prescriptions (ETP).* A research study with consumers who had registered with the three ETP pilot sites indicated that a significant minority liked the convenience of an online repeat prescription service, especially when it was linked to reordering reminders from the pharmacist.[15] Some medicine suppliers have engaged the services of doctors in order to perform online consultations that result in a prescription for a medicine that can then be dispensed and dispatched by mail order.

Prescription medicines are also promoted for sale on the basis of the supply being made with minimal/no intervention from a prescriber. This may target people who wish to circumvent the normal process on the grounds that they would not otherwise be able to receive the medicine, or perhaps that they can streamline their supply without having the inconvenience of visits to a health professional or having to order repeat prescriptions. These products may have specific representations among the public, and the risk of stigma. Medicines commonly promoted include 'lifestyle' products such as prescription medicines for erectile dysfunction, depression/anxiety, and weight loss. This supply route, and its role in inappropriate medicines supply, receives much attention from the popular media and concern from health professionals. But the fact that these routes exist and persist is an indication that consumers perceive barriers in the traditional supply routes, and that those who decide on a particular therapy will pay a premium and accept an element of risk in order to obtain that medicine.

There are also many non-prescription medicines that are offered legitimately for sale through online retailers. The Internet offers small manufacturers and retailers a platform to extend the traditional mail order purchase of food supplements and unlicensed products. The consumer has to determine whether they trust the retailer, and whether the product is safe and relevant for their needs. Finding independent and objective information about complementary medicines

---

* A system by which prescription data is transferred directly from the general practitioner to the pharmacist.

and food supplements can be difficult, since many sites are those of suppliers or enthusiastic supporters.

Licensed medicines are also available for sale through online pharmacies and drugstores. General sales list medicines* can be sold freely by these means. UK pharmacy only medicines† can also be sold, and UK online pharmacies have built a facility into their ordering system to assess whether the medicine is suitable for supply through questions similar to those that would be asked during a normal visit in person to a pharmacy. The Royal Pharmaceutical Society of Great Britain has incorporated guidance into its Code of Ethics for online pharmacies, and provides a fact sheet for pharmacists who wish to provide these services.[16]

Information providers

Portals

Medicines information may be incorporated into a number of different types of consumer website. The sites of the main search engines, huge online 'brands' in their own right, have become community sites that feature information grouped into sections, one of which is usually health (an example is Yahoo™).[17] There is a list of medicines, or groups of medicines, and sites are indexed for those specific headings. The site acts as a portal; it does not author its own information. Thus the perceived expertise of the site to which the consumer is directed may need to be assessed by them, but its trustworthiness may be enhanced by its association with the search engine. Sites can be suggested to Yahoo through an online form and then the editorial site team reviews the content of the suggested site. Those who wish to have their review expedited (seven day maximum) pay a fee for this service.

The NHS and Department of Health

NHS Direct Online is the National Health Service's key initiative in Internet-based provision for consumers. Its initial focus was on decision support for the course of action to take in response to illness by producing a 'Self-Help Guide'. A set of algorithms was developed for this purpose, linked to text information about conditions and brief information on self-care. Consumers can access the information

---

* Medicines available for sale through pharmacies and other outlets, such as supermarkets.

† Medicines that must be sold under the supervision of a pharmacist.

they need using a diagram of the body, clicking on the relevant part, a design feature intended to overcome issues of health literacy in relation to the names of different symptoms and conditions. The site has a Health Encyclopaedia and Common Health Questions.

The National Institute for Health and Clinical Excellence (NICE)[13] website contains clinical guidelines and technology assessments of medicines. Until recently these documents were produced only for health professionals, but a version for patients/carers is now available for some (e.g. heart failure).

The Clinical Knowledge Summaries website[18] comprises guidance on a wide range of conditions designed for use by general practitioners, nurses and pharmacists prescribing in primary care. The site includes a large list of patient information leaflets produced by PRODIGY as well as links to patient organisation websites.

The NICE publishes patient/carer information in association with each of its clinical guidelines. These documents are written in patient-friendly language and summarise the key information (for example, about preferred treatments). However, by their nature they are not detailed and do not contain the evidence about individual treatments. BestTreatments,[19] in contrast, contains the same evidence in its 'patient' section as in its 'doctors' section.

The National Prescribing Centre (NPC)[20] website contains a range of information and resources. These include supporting documents for the practical implementation of prescribing (for example, a guide to good practice in systems for repeat prescribing). Some parts of the site are public access and others are password-protected and intended for NHS users (for example, prescribing and pharmaceutical advisers).

Apart from NHS information at a national level, there is scope for individual NHS trusts to host their own information about medicines for their local patients. The Tayside Diabetes Network[21] has a series of patient information leaflets, including guides to the use of insulin. Moorfield's Eye Hospital has an 'eye health' section within its institutional site[22] that describes some of the principal treatments for common eye conditions under its care. Again, the expertise and trustworthiness of this information from a NHS trust is likely to be high, and the empathy increased as patients may feel a strong sense of identification with the institution responsible for their own care.

The Medicines and Healthcare Products Regulatory Agency (MHRA)[23] is responsible for the licensing of medicines, for changes in the legal status of medicines and for pharmacovigilance once medicines are prescribed. Its website contains current consultation documents (for example, when it is proposed that a medicine should be reclassified from prescription only to pharmacy medicine status) and updates on important medicines safety information.

Professional bodies

The Royal Pharmaceutical Society and British Medical Association jointly produce the twice-yearly *British National Formulary* which is available online as eBNF (www.bnf.org).[24] Intended for prescribers, the *BNF* provides a summary of all medicines available in the UK in the context of their therapeutic use. A recent addition is the BNF-C (bnfc.org),[25] in the same format but specialising in information about children's medicines.

The Royal Pharmaceutical Society has recently revised its website and has created a double-entry point for its professional members and for the public. One section relates to individuals' questions about their own medicines, and the RPSGB has listed a number of websites that it considers credible for medicines information.[26]

Patient organisations and charities

Self-help organisation sites, responding to the needs of patients with a defined condition, or range of conditions, also provide overviews, and sometimes detailed information, about the medicine options for those conditions (an example is the National Endometriosis Society[27]). The empathy of these sites could be high for people who identify with the condition/s featured. The expertise of these sites may be determined by the authorship of the materials they produce: a national association that holds meetings and has a membership is likely to be perceived as more trustworthy than information from an isolated sufferer. The DiPEx (Directory of Patient Experience)[28] charity site contains text, video and audio content on a wide range of conditions and their treatment. The content is sourced from interviews conducted with patients and is thus presented in patients' own words. The site contains a detailed explanation of its methods of generating content, its funding policy (it does not accept funding from pharmaceutical companies) and its sources of expertise. The site's empathy, expertise and trustworthiness are likely to be high. NetDoctor provides a Medicines Encyclopaedia, compiled by pharmacists, and including information about uses and side effects written in lay language.[29]

The geographical origin of medicines information may not always be obvious to consumers. This is particularly relevant when considering online medicines information from manufacturers. Pharmaceutical companies are prohibited from placing information about prescription-only medicines on their European websites. A search for such a medicine may therefore yield information from another country's site, where different regulations apply. For example, if a search engine query for 'Ventolin' is restricted to UK sites, the first entries are from the Electronic Medicines Compendium's 'Medicine Guides'[30] and no manufacturer links are listed. If this restriction is lifted, the first entry is the US site 'ventolin.com', followed by the site of the manufacturer Glaxo SmithKline 'gsk.com'. The expertise of these information sources is likely to be regarded highly. Consumers may, however, be sceptical of the commercial nature of pharmaceutical companies. Empathy and trustworthiness may therefore be lower.

Some pharmaceutical companies have been supporting self-help groups, including their websites, perhaps recognising the strong empathy and trust that they engender in those with the featured condition. An editorial by Andrew Herxheimer in the *BMJ* in May 2003 cited the example of the Lymphoma Association and their relationship with Roche.[31] The Association's portal[32] at that time had several sites, including one for professionals and one for the public. Health professionals were asked to register with the site, leading to a reference to an educational grant from Roche products. The consumer site was freely accessible and had no declared affiliation to Roche, except in the 'disclaimer' part of the site.

A website where patients can access the same information as prescribers, BestTreatments[19] is also available. The content is based on systematic reviews of clinical trials published in *Clinical Evidence*,[33] written in a consumer-friendly style and with additional information about the condition.

The mediators

The Internet has the potential to facilitate public access to medicines information hitherto only available through specialist publications and from professionals. Potential advantages for the public include 24-hour private access, rapidly updated information, a choice of information providers, and the ability to print out and keep relevant information for future use. Previous delineation of medicines information sources, such as books, for professionals or consumers, has diminished on the Internet. Although online information providers may still focus on one or other of these groups, the reality is that most sites are available to both. Some providers have acknowledged this by offering separate sections tailored to the perceived needs of different groups, but research is lacking as to whether either group 'strays' into the other's territory.

The challenges
Credibility and trust

These challenges already face medicine consumers. Traditional mass media provide medicines information in a variety of formats (e.g. editorial content, advertisements, and news stories), from an extensive range of information providers (e.g. manufacturers, 'celebrity doctors', and health correspondents). The additional challenge with online information, however, is that the Internet is not a mature medium, and there is no equivalent heritage of 'broadsheet-tabloid' differentiation that helps consumers to judge the credibility of the information source. Tony Delamothe has asserted that information seekers use brands to discriminate between sources in other media such as newspapers.[34] The presence of online information sources that are well-known 'offline' may help as signposts for consumers and professionals alike.

With increased access, the consumer medicines information seeker takes on extra challenges and responsibilities. They may need to be able to spell the name of the medicine correctly to initiate a meaningful online search. They have to develop criteria and search strategies that will help them to locate relevant and credible information (formerly 'filtered' for them by professionals). They must learn to distinguish promotional material from evidence-based information, and evaluate the consequences of relying upon online information in a potentially high-risk health decision.

Several studies have explored how consumers use the Internet, through observation and focus groups. Peterson et al.[35] found in Australia that all her focus group participants used a search engine for their query, typing in the generic or brand name directly. The sophistication of these searches differed. Some users typed medicine names in as the web address (URL). The authors concluded that their respondents saw the Internet as an important information source, but that their search skills varied widely and they did not consciously think about how they selected medicines information from the search results that they obtained. Hansen *et al.*[36] observed US adolescents using the Internet to achieve pre-defined tasks, and cited spelling proficiency, overall search strategy and the number of pages visited within a site as important determinants of success.

Quality of Internet sites

Studies of the quality of available information on the Internet have raised questions about the accuracy and currency of content (see for example, Impiccatore *et al.*[37]). One response from clinicians has been a call for 'kitemarking' of 'approved' sites but as Tann points out, 'Internet censorship is not only difficult but also, in all probability, counter-productive'.[38]

There seems to be much anxiety among health professionals and policymakers about the potential for the Internet to misinform patients.[39,40] This is manifested by numerous academic papers regarding the quality of web-based information about subjects as diverse as depression and the treatment of fever in children.[41, 42] Commentators have advocated and implemented a range of quality marking systems,[43] and the World Health Organization has – unsuccessfully – sought a '.health' suffix on Web addresses for sites that meet certain quality criteria.[44]

Others have cited the impracticality of the task and the need to resist imposition of medical dominance on health information.[34,45] The central question seems to be whose definition of 'quality' is valid, and it may be argued that this validity varies according to the nature of the search. Why should an account of a patient's experience on a specific medicine be any less useful to a user with a problem than a Cochrane systematic review?

The European Council supported an initiative to develop a core set of 'Quality Criteria for Health related Websites'.[46] There were eight categories of criteria: transparency and honesty; authority; privacy and data protection; updating of information; accountability; responsible partnering; editorial policy; and accessibility. The last category includes guidelines on physical accessibility, general 'findability', searchability, readability and usability. There is recognised good practice in sites stating their policies on these issues. In relation to medicines there is considerable debate about pharmaceutical company funding of, for example, sites of patient support groups.[47]

The Health On the Net Foundation (HON),[48] created in 1995, is a not-for-profit non-governmental organisation under the aegis of the Direction Générale de la Santé Département de l'Action Sociale et de Santé (DASS-République et canton de Genève, Switzerland). HON's mission is to guide laypersons or non-medical users and medical practitioners to useful and reliable online medical and health information. HON provides leadership in setting ethical standards for website developers.

Interestingly, Nettleton *et al.*[49] believe that a consensus is naturally emerging between lay use of the Internet and the accepted biomedical definition of 'good quality' online health information.

The future
Effects of consumer Internet use on consultations with health professionals

In the past health professionals were able to act as 'filters', controlling the flow of information. Access to the Internet has been the biggest single challenge to professionals' traditional power based on the asymmetry of knowledge and information.

Possible outcomes of accessing Internet-based medicines information for consumers include:

- discussing the information with a health professional
- challenging a health professional's treatment recommendation
- deciding not to use/take a medicine
- changing the way a health issue is managed
- buying a medicine online
- buying a medicine from a pharmacy or other outlet.

Only 16% of Australian consumers who accessed health information from the Internet subsequently discussed it with their doctor or pharmacist.[1] The effects on consultations thus may be direct or indirect. Theoretically, better informed consumers will be more able to participate in consultations with health professionals. In turn health professionals will need to respond to the different information that consumers bring to the discussion.

In Tann's study of psychiatrists 30% believed that clients' use of the Internet led to a greater partnership with clients.[38] Perceived advantages of client use of the Internet were informing clients about their illness, giving ownership/control, enabling access to support groups and providing a sense of partnership. Three categories of negative effects of Internet use emerged: the quality of information obtained, changed patient/carer expectations, and changed clinician/patient/carer relationships.

Tann notes that her data 'suggest[s] that patients are not always willing to reveal their Internet exploration of therapy alternatives unless the clinician first indicates a willingness to discuss them'.

The effect of the Internet on the doctor-patient relationship is becoming a major research theme in its own right.[50] Murray *et al.*[7] found that prescribers granted inappropriate requests from patients who came with Internet information, possibly because they did not want to damage the doctor-patient relationship. Most physicians felt that the patient's use of Internet information was beneficial or neutral to the consultation.

Results from the first 'Health Information National Trends Survey' in the US suggest that almost half of their adult sample went to the Internet for information before visiting their doctor,[51] confirming an increasing trend.

Realising the potential for users with special needs

It is notable that the potential of the Internet to present information in ways that would help people with sensory impairment or low literacy has not yet been fully realised. Many medicines information sites are electronic recreations of text in printed form. 'Hypertext' that takes a user from one page to another can be very helpful in order to explain medical jargon or jump to relevant related sections. This is used extensively in sites such as the eBNF and Best Treatments.

The use of complementary graphics and illustrations, however, is low. In 2002 the UK Government, through the Office of the e-Envoy, issued a quality framework for UK Government website design.[52] The guidelines highlight that the website must, by law, be accessible to the disabled. The challenge with online information seems to be providing material that can be accessed by the range of web browsers and computers that the public have, whilst including graphics and interactive features. The US Department for Health and Human Services compiled a site called 'usability.gov', where research into website design informs a set of guidelines.[53] Examples of their tools for web designers to broaden access include colour blindness simulation drivers and text-only browsers that indicate how sites would sound to a speech user.

The US National Institute on Ageing and National Library of

Medicine has created a site called 'NIH Senior Health',[54] which uses technology to assist older people through the site. This technology includes a setting for larger text, speech browsing, and high contrast pages. Topics include treatments for older people's conditions, such as arthritis.

Other users are challenged by this text-driven medium. The US Children's Partnership has undertaken research with low income and underserved Americans, including people with low literacy and those who speak English as a second language, and has found that their general needs are:[55]

- practical information focusing on the local community, at a basic literacy level
- material in multiple languages
- spaces for ethnic and cultural interests
- interfaces and content suitable for people with disabilities
- easier searching
- coaches to guide them.

It makes sense that these principles would help to inform our underserved populations about their medicines, such as culturally sensitive information about medicine-taking and religious beliefs. The idea of coaches is also consistent with a notion of health professionals as navigators.

Interactive and individualised medicines information

One example of innovation on the Internet for medicines information is the 'Medicines Information Project' (MIP), promoted by the Medicines Partnership and compiled by Datapharm Communications.[56] MIP is steered by a collaborative where patient groups, professionals, the National Patient Safety Agency (NPSA) and the Department of Health are all represented. One of the classic criticisms of existing patient information leaflets with medicines is the lack of specificity and tailoring of advice; for example, information about pregnancy and breast-feeding is redundant for men. The 'Medicine Guide' initiative enables an individual to insert details of their gender and edits the guide accordingly. The text is enhanced by hypertext and by another form of link where letting the mouse hover above the word produces a glossary box with a short alternative definition of the medical word. These guides cover a range of conditions and medicines and more are planned.

Changing usage of medicines information

This chapter started by identifying the four broad categories of users of online health information. To conclude this chapter these groups are reconsidered with particular reference to likely future developments.

Consumers

Consumer use of the Internet will almost certainly continue to increase. Information available about medicines will become more personalised. The information used to achieve this personalisation may be stored securely on sites such as My NHS HealthSpace so that users do not have to answer online surveys each time. Information for those with special needs (disability and low literacy) will develop.

Practitioner/adviser

It has been suggested that clinicians 'will increasingly act as information guides, rather than information resources'.[57] Health professionals will need to be better-prepared to discuss information their clients and carers have obtained from the Internet.

Prescriber

The advent of the EHR (electronic health record) will enable the prescriber to review many different aspects of the patient's health, including adherence through links to dispensing records and factors affecting concordance such as a patient's social circumstances (presence of a carer etc.). Integrated decision support systems and guidelines will drive higher prescribing quality.

Policymakers/resource allocators

As work progresses on the NHS information strategy, 'Information for Health', the potential for policymakers to extract population medicine use statistics and epidemiological information from local health communities will be realised. This will enable more accurate planning, allocation and monitoring of resources. The interplay between individual medicine use and that of the population will be more dynamically and usefully mapped.

Conclusion

The Internet and online health information are becoming increasingly established in healthcare as in other walks of life. It is important that the many advantages of this are maximised through education of the public and of professionals. To maintain safety and minimise risk the supply of medicines via the Internet needs appropriate regulation and public education is key.

References

1. Bessell TL, Silagy C, Anderson JN, Hiller JE, Sansom LN. Prevalence of South Australia's online health seekers. *Aust & NZ J Pub Health* 2002; **26**(2): 170–3.
2. Brodie M, Flournoy RE, Altman DE, Blendon RJ, Benson JM, Rosenbaum MD. Health information, the internet, and the digital divide. *Health Affairs 2000*; **19**: 255–65.
3. Zeng QT, Kogan S, Plovnick RM, Crowell J, Lacroix EM, Greenes RA. Positive attitudes and failed queries: an exploration of the conundrums of health information retrieval. *Int J Med Inf* 2004; **73**(1): 45–55.
4. Department of Health. Public attitudes to self care – Baseline survey. 2005.
5. McColl A, Smith H, White P, Field J. General practitioners' perceptions of the route to evidence-based medicine: a questionnaire survey. *BMJ* 1998; **316**: 361–5.
6. Estabrooks CA, O'Leary KA, Ricker KL, Humphrey CK. The internet and access to evidence: how are nurses positioned? *J Advanced Nurs* 2003; **42**(1): 73–81.
7. Murray E, Lo B, Pollack L, Donelan K, Catania J, Lee K, Zapert K, Turner R. The impact of health information on the Internet on health care and the physician-patient relationship: National US survey among 1050 US physicians. *JMIR* 2003; **5**(3): e17.
8. Cost Effectiveness and Resource Allocation (online journal). Ed: Evans, D. Available at http://www.resource-allocation.com/info/about/ (accessed 14 August 2007).
9. National Electronic Library for Health. http://www.nelh.nhs.uk/. National Library for Health. http://www.library.nhs.uk/
10. Cunningham SM. Perceived Risk and Brand Loyalty. In: Cox DF, editor. *Risk Taking and Information Handling in Consumer Behaviour.* Boston: Harvard University; 1967: 507–23.
11. Gore P, Madhavan S. Credibility of the sources of information for non-prescription medicines. *J Soc Admin Pharm* 1993; **10**(3): 109–22.
12. http://www.nhsdirect.nhs.uk
13. National Institute for Health and Clinical Evidence. http://www.nice.org.uk
14. National Electronic Library for Medicines. http://www.nelm.nhs.uk
15. Phul S, Cooper SL, Cantrill JA. Pharmacy services and patient choice: insights into differences between patient groups. *IJPP* 2003; **11**: 233–42.

16. Professional Standards and Guidance for Internet Pharmacy Services http://www.rpsgb.org/pdfs/coepsgintpharm.pdf (accessed 14 August 2007).
17. http://uk.dir.yahoo.com/Health/ (Yahoo health and medicines).
18. Clinical Knowledge Summaries. http://www.cks.library.nhs.uk
19. http://www.besttreatments.co.uk
20. National Prescribing Centre. http://www.npc.co.uk
21. http://www.diabetes-healthnet.ac.uk/ (Tayside Diabetes Clinical Network).
22. http://www.moorfields.org.uk/EyeHealth (Moorfields Eye Hospital).
23. http://www.mhra.gov.uk/ (Medicines and Healthcare Products Regulatory Agency).
24. http://www.bnf.org/ (BNF).
25. BNF for Children. http://www.bnfc.nhs.uk/bnfc/
26. RPSGB. http://www.rpsgb.org
27. http://www.endo.org.uk/ (National Endometriosis Society).
28. Dipex. http://www.dipex.org
29. http://www.netdoctor.co.uk/ (Medicines Encyclopaedia).
30. Electronic Medicines Compendium.
31. Herxheimer A. Relationships between the pharmaceutical industry and patients' organisations. *BMJ* 2003; **326**: 1208–10.
32. http://www.lymphoma.org.uk/ (Lymphoma Association).
33. Clinical Evidence. http://www.clinicalevidence.com
34. Delamothe T. Quality of websites: kitemarking the west wind. *BMJ* 2000; **321**: 843–4.
35. Peterson G, Aslani P, Williams KA. How do consumers search for and appraise information on medicines on the internet? A qualitative study using focus groups. *JMIR* 2003; **5**(4): e33.
36. Hansen DL, Derry HA, Resnick PJ, Richardson CR. Adolescents searching for health information on the internet: an observational study. *JMIR* 2003; **5**(4): e25.
37. Impiccatore P, Pandolfini C, Casella N, Bonati M. Reliability of health information for the public on the world wide web: a systematic survey of advice on managing fever in children at home. *BMJ* 1997; **314**: 1875–8.
38. Tann J, Platts A, Welch S, Allen J. Patient Power? Medical perspectives on patient use of the internet. *Prometheus* 2003; **21**(2): 145–60.
39. Arunachalam S. Assuring quality and relevance of internet information in the real world. *BMJ* 1998; **317**: 1501–02.
40. Griffiths KM, Christensen H. Quality of web based information on treatment of depression: cross sectional survey. *BMJ* 2000; **321**: 1511–15.
41. Bonati M, Impicciatore P, Pandolfini C. Quality on the internet. *BMJ* 1998; **317**: 1501.
42. Fallis D, Fricke M. Indicators of accuracy of consumer health information on the internet: a study of indicators relating to information for managing fever in children in the home. *JAMIA* 2002; **9**(1): 73–9.

43. Eysenbach G, Diepgen TL. Towards quality management of medical information on the internet: evaluation, labelling, and filtering of information. *BMJ* 1998; **317**: 1496–502.

44. Anonymous. WHO bid to regulate health sites. BBC Health News, 13 November 2000. Available at http://news.bbc.co.uk/1/hi/health/1021390.stm (accessed 14 August 2007).

45. Kendall L. *The Future Patient.* London: IPPR; 2001.

46. Commission of the European Communities, Brussels. EEurope 2002: Quality Criteria for Health related Websites. *J Medical Internet Research* 2002; **4**(3): e15. http://www.jmir.org/2002/3/e15/ (accessed 14 August 2007).

47. Patient Groups Special: Swallowing the best advice? http://www.new scientist.com/article.ns?id=mg19225755.100&feedId=us_rss20

48. http://www.hon.ch/ (Health on the Net Foundation).

49. Nettleton S, Burrows R, O'Malley L. The mundane realities of the everyday lay use of the internet for health, and their consequences for media convergence. *Sociol Health Illn* 2005; **27**(7): 972–92.

50. Gerber BS, Eiser AR. The patient-physician relationship in the Internet Age: Future prospects and the research agenda. *JMIR* 2001; **3**(2): e15. Available at http://www.jmir.org/2001/2/e15/ (accessed 14 August 2007).

51. Hesse BW, Nelson DE, Kreps GL, Croyle RT, Arora NK, Rimer BK, Viswanath K. Trust and sources of health information: the impact of the internet and its implications for health care providers: findings from the first Health Information National Trends Survey. *Arch Intern Med* 2005; **165**(22): 2618–24.

52. Cabinet Office. Office of the e-Envoy: Web Guidelines. Available at: http://archive.cabinetoffice.gov.uk/e-envoy/index-content.htm (NB: no www prefix).

53. US Department of Health and Human Services. Research-based Web Design and Usability Guidelines. Usability.gov. Available at: http://usability.gov/guidelines/guidelines_notice.html (accessed 14 August 2007).

54. National Institutes of Health. NIHSeniorHealth.gov. Last updated: 23 October 2003. Available at: http://nihseniorhealth.gov/ (accessed 14 August 2007).

55. Children's Partnership. Online Content for Low Income and Underserved Americans: 2002 Update. Available at http://www.childrenspartnership.org/AM/Template.cfm?Section=Case_Study_Online_Content (accessed 14 August 2007).

56. Datapharm Communications Limited. About the Medicines Information Partnership (MIP). Available at: http://www.medicines.org.uk/medguides.aspx (accessed 14 August 2007).

57. Glode LM. Challenges and opportunities of the internet for medical oncology. *J Clinical Oncology* 1996; **14**(7): 2181–6

6 Pharmacoepidemiology, public health and pharmacy

ROGER WALKER

This chapter defines pharmacoepidemiology, outlines the scope of epidemiological studies, and provides examples of their application to monitoring drug use.

Introduction

Pharmacoepidemiology is best defined as the study of the utilisation and effects, whether beneficial or adverse, of drugs in large numbers of individuals. It is a discipline often described as one that spans both clinical pharmacology and epidemiology and has evolved from the need to evaluate the unintended effects of drugs following their introduction into clinical practice. Increasingly it is a core discipline of pharmacy and public health as the use of drugs is mapped across a given population and evidence of appropriate use, inappropriate use or inequalities gathered.

Probably the first formal pharmacoepidemiological studies were those that investigated a link between the use of a drug and an adverse reaction. The best known of these occurred in the late 1950s and early 1960s when the link between thalidomide, marketed as a sedative and hypnotic, and babies born with a congenital malformation of the limbs known as phocomelia, were investigated. In recent years pharmacoepidemiology has contributed to public health by identifying rare adverse effects, promoting evidence-based prescribing practice, uncovering questionable prescribing patterns and highlighting inequalities in disease management.

Scope of pharmacoepidemiology

Pharmacoepidemiological studies play a part in almost every aspect of medicine use from regulation to clinical practice, with the regulatory process providing the original rationale for undertaking such studies. It is easy to understand why this is the case when drug development is examined. In most countries the drug approval process involves laboratory, animal and human testing with testing in humans involving three phases:

Phase I: trials in volunteers to determine safe dosage range, pharmacokinetics and toxicity

Phase II: trials in small numbers of closely monitored patients to evaluate safety, efficacy and optimal dosing

Phase III: trials in 500 to 3000 patients to evaluate safety, efficacy and dosing.

It is not unknown for serious adverse reactions to go undetected during pre-market testing because these studies typically involve small numbers of patients, are of short duration, and recruit individuals from selected populations. As a consequence these pre-marketing studies poorly reflect use in normal clinical practice where greater numbers of patients, often with comorbities and other concomitant medications, are exposed to the drug in an uncontrolled environment, and rare or serious side effects may be revealed. Postmarketing pharmacoepidemiological studies are therefore used to generate data to complement that collected during pre-market testing. The process of monitoring medicines to identify unrecognised adverse effects, changes in the patterns of adverse effects and the risks and benefits of use is often referred to as pharmacovigilance.[1] It is recognised as a subspecialty within pharmacoepidemiology, and is described in more detail in Chapter 9.

The continuous, postmarketing monitoring of the safe use of medicinal products is a key area for pharmacovigilance and is important to the protection of public health. Within the European Economic Area (EEA), legislation is in place to ensure that national competent authorities, marketing authorisation holders, applicants and sponsors of clinical trials collect, collate and exchange data on adverse drug reactions. This is facilitated by EudraVigilance, the European data-processing network and management system that was launched in December 2001. From May 2004 the sponsors of all clinical trials in the EEA must ensure all relevant information about suspected unexpected serious adverse reactions (SUSARs) are reported and all SUSARs sent electronically to the EudraVigilance clinical trials module.[1]

In the specific case of orphan drugs there is a more liberal approach to the granting of marketing authorisation and consequently a greater need for postmarketing surveillance. Orphan drug status is conferred on those medicines used to treat disorders with a prevalence of less than 5 per 10000. This status also confers market exclusivity to encourage research into treatments for rare diseases. It is the simplest and quickest way to place a medicinal product on the market throughout the EEA. The available evidence base may be poorer than for more traditional new drugs because clinical trials are difficult to conduct in rare diseases. As a consequence, licensing bodies such as the European Agency for the Evaluation of Medical Products (EMEA) may request postmarketing epidemiological studies. Other benefits of collecting pharmacoepidemiological data include the monitoring and evaluation of drug safety, monitoring patterns of drug use, estimating risk or testing other hypotheses.

From the above it can be seen that pharmacoepidemiology is the science that underpins postmarketing drug surveillance. It utilises a variety of designs and data sources and can generate results more rapidly than controlled trials albeit with significant limitations. The traditional approach to undertaking pharmacoepidemiological studies will be outlined in the next section and followed by examples of use in practice.

Types of study

In their simplest form pharmacoepidemiological studies can be classified as either experimental or observational (*see* Table 6.1).

The majority of studies are observational and the variable under study, for example the drug treatment, is not controlled. The exception to this is the randomised controlled trial, although this is artificial and may deny active treatment to individuals in one arm of the study who, for example, receive a placebo.

Study design

As well as the two broad types of study, there are also different study designs. A brief overview of some examples of the advantages and disadvantages of the different study designs are outlined in Table 6.2. The study designs are described briefly below, and are also referred to in Chapter 3.

TABLE 6.1 Examples of studies that could be used to test the hypothesis that exposure to a drug is associated with a specific adverse effect

TYPE OF STUDY	COMMENT
Experimental	
Laboratory experiment	Randomised allocation to treatment with drug
	Exposure to drug and environment can be controlled
Field experiment	Randomised allocation to treatment with drug
	Limited control of exposure to drug and environment
Analytic observational	
Cross-sectional	Sampling of population without prior knowledge of exposure to drug or adverse reaction status
Case-control	Sampling of population based on adverse reaction status
Cohort	Sampling of population based on knowledge of exposure to drug

Randomised controlled trial

Randomised controlled trials are often considered the gold standard of study designs. Typically a given treatment is compared with one or more alternate treatments or with no treatment at all (placebo). The key methodological aspect is that equal numbers of participants are randomly allocated to each treatment. To further minimise the chance of bias the trial is carried out double blind. This involves both the doctor/investigator and the patient being unaware of the group to which the patient has been allocated. It is usual to calculate in advance the number of participants required to be recruited to show a significant difference between the treatment arms. When that number of individuals have been exposed to the treatments the outcomes in each group are compared.

Case report

Case reports describe the outcome of exposure of an individual patient to a drug and can be useful to indicate the beneficial and/or intended effect or adverse effect of a drug. Where there are indications that a drug may be associated with an untoward effect it is theoretically possible to re-challenge with the suspected agent. In practical terms this approach is often unacceptable since it may re-expose the patient to a serious adverse effect.

TABLE 6.2 Example of advantages and disadvantages associated with different types of pharmacoepidemiological study

STUDY DESIGN	ADVANTAGES	DISADVANTAGES
Randomised clinical trial	Accepted robust design	Expensive
	Controls for unknowns and confounders	Contrived
		Ethical issues e.g. placebo group denied active treatment
Case report	Low cost	No indication of incidence
	Generates hypothesis	
	De-challenge/re-challenge establishes causality	
Case series	Indicates incidence	No control group
		Unable to test hypothesis
Time trend	Undertaken rapidly	Group analysis
		Cause undetermined
		No control for confounding issues
Case control	Can study uncommon problems in small populations	Bias of subjects when reliant on recall
	Low cost	
	Undertaken rapidly	
Cohort study	Prospective or retrospective	Expensive
	Ideal for studies of single exposure	May require large sample size
	No control group required	Long time required for prospective studies

Case series

Case series provide reports of outcome in a group of patients exposed to a given drug. Case series are useful for quantifying the incidence of an event related to the drug or identifying whether it occurs when a population larger than that used in pre-marketing studies is exposed to it. Case series do not permit establishment of causality because there is no control group.

Time trend

When studying time or secular trends a relationship between exposure to a drug and a presumed effect can be explored. An example of this could be where drug exposure is compared with the change in incidence of a given medical condition in various sectors of the population.

Case control

In a case control study the exposure of a group of patients in whom a disease or disorder has developed is compared to that of a control group without the problem. These studies are useful in analysing cases with many alternative causes for a disorder and can also be used to quantify risk. Unlike cohort studies, matching does not eradicate confounding and is normally retrospective after cases have developed the disease or other characteristic under study. Unfortunately, case control studies are very susceptible to bias that can arise from the selection of the actual cases and controls or the method of data collection. For example, individuals who are taking regular medication will probably have more contact with their doctor and this will thereby increase the likelihood that any new mild or asymptomatic disorder is diagnosed and create a spurious relationship between medication and the mild disorder.

Cohort

Cohort studies involve groups (cohorts) of individuals with defined characteristics. They are normally followed prospectively over a fixed period of time with the outcome in the different cohorts compared, e.g. incidence of breast cancer in users of hormone replacement therapy compared to incidence in women who have not used hormone replacement therapy.[2] Cohort studies have also been used to investigate the relationship between the use of calcium channel blockers and risk of suicide.[3] Here 617 subjects (18%) were classified as users of calcium channel blockers and 2780 (82%) as non-users. The risk of suicide for those receiving a calcium channel blocker compared to other antihypertensive medication was calculated after adjustment for differences in age and sex. Cohort studies are particularly poor at assessing efficacy and when studies are undertaken over several years there may need to be allowances for the ageing of study participants.

Pragmatic studies

To identify whether the use of a drug in a given population is associated with a particular positive or negative outcome is a common question. Such questions lend themselves to a variety of study designs, such as those discussed above. However, in practice many questions arise about the routine use of medicines which need to be answered quickly, and this is often done utilising routinely available prescribing or dispensing data. The following are typical examples.

- Do patterns of medicine use reflect implementation of national guidelines?
- Is the use of antibiotics declining in a given population?
- Are some prescribers more likely than others to prescribe new drugs?
- Are prescribing patterns consistent with disease prevalence?
- Does deprivation impact on medicine use?
- Is the use of a given medicine associated with an adverse event?

Given the widespread availability of comprehensive dispensing data in the United Kingdom (*see also* Chapters 1 and 7), created as a consequence of the need to remunerate pharmacies for supplying prescribed medicines as part of the National Health Service, many use this data to answer the questions posed above. Others attempt to use dispensing data to answer more complex questions or monitor prescribing performance and consequently generate answers that may be misleading if the limitations of dispensing data, and the factors that create bias and confounding, are not clearly understood.

Monitoring prescribing performance

Typically the monitoring of prescribing performance has focused on the volume and cost of prescribing and expenditure against a budget. Dispensing data, which contains the number of items, quantity and cost of a given product dispensed is more than adequate to answer such questions. However, with attempts to monitor the quality and appropriateness of prescribing, routine dispensing data has many limitations. Attempts to circumvent this have emerged such as the collection of data on the patient list size of each general medical practice to allow comparators such as items prescribed per patient, cost per patient and cost per item to be developed. The impact of age and the fact that elderly patients generally receive more prescribed medicines has led to the development of the prescribing unit (PU), the more refined age, sex, temporary resident originated prescribing unit (ASTRO-PU) and the specific therapeutic age-sex related prescribing unit (STAR-PU) comparator. Others have tried to standardise the actual volume prescribed by different prescribers by utilising defined daily doses (DDDs) or average daily quantities (ADQ).

Prescribing unit (PU)

It has been long recognised that elderly patients receive more medication than their younger counterparts. For example, two medical practices with the same list size and in the same area, but one having a predominantly elderly population, will have prescribing levels that reflect the greater number of elderly subjects. They also need a prescribing budget to support this. To calculate this a weighting factor is used to reflect the greater need of elderly patients for medication. Patients under 65 years of age and temporary residents count as one prescribing unit (PU) and patients aged 65 or over count as three PUs.

Age, sex, temporary resident originated prescribing unit (ASTRO-PU)

The PU is a very simple weighting factor and has been refined so that the effect of age, sex and the number of temporary residents on a practice's prescribing budget can be better predicted. The age, sex, temporary resident originated prescribing unit (ASTRO-PU) is based on cost rather than the number of prescription items and is useful for comparing overall costs of prescribing between practices or groups of practices.

Specific therapeutic age-sex related prescribing units (STAR-PUs)

Specific therapeutic age-sex related prescribing units (STAR-PUs) were developed[4] as a weighting to more accurately reflect the influence of patient age and sex on prescribing costs within a therapeutic group, e.g. cardiovascular drugs, or a specific therapeutic class, e.g. lipid lowering agents. For example, the STAR-PU weighting for lipid lowering agents reflects their relative higher use in a population comprising males aged 45 to 74 years compared to younger patients or females of a similar age. These are shown in Table 6.3.

Although the shift from cost and item comparators to STAR-PUs permits a more elegant analysis and clearly aids comparison between practices or across a defined population, STAR-PUs give little indication of appropriateness of use in the individual patient, do not reflect whether the medicine was taken, may vary markedly between given populations (as may PUs and ASTRO-PUs) and require updating at regular intervals to reflect changes in prescribing or the publication of national guidelines.

Two other values have been developed to help address this, the defined daily dose and the average daily quantity.

TABLE 6.3 Example of STAR-PU weightings for age and gender for lipid lowering agents

AGE GROUP	MALE	FEMALE
0–4	0	0
5–14	0	0
15–24	0	0
25–34	0.3	0.2
35–44	2.6	0.7
45–54	10.6	3.4
55–64	25.1	12.6
65–74	30.4	24.2

Defined daily dose (DDD)

In terms of volume of medicines dispensed, a prescription item is not a good indicator of volume. Although the majority of items on prescriptions are for a 28 day period a significant minority are not and could also be prescribed in any one of a number of dose permutations. To overcome these problems the World Health Organization devised and maintains a list of defined daily doses (DDD) for each drug. Each drug is allocated a value for its DDD based on the average, daily maintenance dose used for its main indication in adults. The DDD for drugs with a similar indication are deemed to be functionally equivalent and can be added together. It must be remembered, however, that DDDs are a unit of measure and may not be a real dose. DDDs are also discussed in more detail in Chapter 7.

Average daily quantity (ADQ)

The values for DDDs are based on international prescribing habits and, as a consequence, may not reflect use in a particular country. In

England a set of values which have become known as average daily quantities (ADQs) have been defined by the prescribing support unit (available at http://www.ic.nhs.uk/psu/) to permit a more accurate analysis and comparison of prescribing in primary care in England. Like DDDs, ADQs are not recommended doses but analytical units that aid comparisons.

Overall there is need for caution when using prescribing comparators whether PUs, ASTRO-PUs or STAR-PUs. They should be used to improve the quality and effectiveness of prescribing and not solely to reduce costs. It has been fashionable in some quarters to equate good prescribers with those who are conservative and limit the volume of drugs prescribed and restrict their use of new and expensive drugs. Clearly this may be inappropriate[5] particularly when there is evidence of benefit and where limiting use may deny patients access to effective therapy. In addition, the use of prescribing comparators must not create a perverse incentive whereby a practice can appear to improve performance as measured by the indicator without improving their clinical management of the patient.

It has been identified[6] that the decision to prescribe a new drug

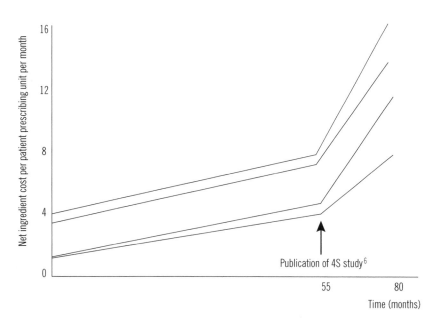

FIGURE 6.1 Each line indicates prescribing of lipid lowering drugs in general practice in one of four health authorities from 1990 to 1996. 4S indicates publication of Scandinavian simvastatin survival study

is not simply related to biomedical evaluation and critical appraisal but more to the mode of exposure to pharmacological information and social influences on decision making. Nevertheless monitoring prescribing patterns and changes in prescribing can be useful. For example, a time trend analysis[7] of lipid prescribing patterns in four health authorities (Figure 6.1) demonstrated the impact of publication of the landmark 4S study[8] on the prescribing of lipid lowering agents. Others[9] have shown that socioeconomic factors, patient's attitudes and demographic differences between and within regions explain prescribing variation, none of which can be readily evaluated using prescribing data.

Medical practice research databases

Regardless of how intricate the manipulation of prescribing data, or how complex the statistical analysis undertaken, there are inherent limitations to prescribing data that restrict use to observational epidemiology. Despite ever larger and increasingly comprehensive computerised healthcare data resources as described in Chapter 7, prescription data only permits comparisons of prescribing patterns between defined populations. The full power of pharmacoepidemiological methods cannot be utilised unless prescription details are linked to patient details. Most European countries have populations covered by universal healthcare systems with the UK, Netherlands, Italy and the Nordic countries having particularly well-developed systems. One of the most widely used databases for pharmacoepidemiological research has been the General Practice Research Database (GPRD) in the UK. It has been used in more than 200 peer reviewed, original articles and has a quarterly, updated bibliography of research publications available.[10]

After a period of data entry and quality control training the general medical practitioners supporting the GPRD enter the necessary medical information into their practice computer. The required data input includes demographics, details of every general practitioner's consultation, a summary of hospital specialists' clinical notes and hospital letters, results of laboratory tests and a free text section. Prescriptions, including dosage instructions, are issued directly from the computer and thus ensure a complete record. Around 1500 general practitioners enter data covering a population of approximately 3 million across all age bands. Since the early 1990s most practices participating in the GPRD have been providing data of a quality suitable for drug research. The GPRD is the largest computerised database in the world containing more than 35 million patient years of anonymised, longitudinal patient records. Other sizeable primary care databases have emerged in the UK and across mainland Europe and North America but few challenge the GPRD for its tried and tested quality.

TABLE 6.4 Identified limitations of published observational epidemiological studies

- Participant selection process, e.g. information on exclusions and refusals often lacks details.
- Quality of data collected and problems therein are often insufficiently described.
- Some studies are too small and prone to exaggerated claims, while few give power calculations to justify their size.
- Quantitative exposure variables are commonly grouped into ordered categories, but few state the rationale for choice of grouping and analyses.
- Terminology for estimates of association, e.g. relative risk, is used inconsistently.
- Confidence intervals are in appropriate widespread use but presented excessively in some articles.
- P values are used sparingly but there is a tendency to over-interpret arbitrary cut-offs such as $P < 0.05$.
- The selection of and adjustment for potential confounders needs greater clarity, consistency and explanation.
- Subgroup analyses to identify effect modifiers mostly lack appropriate methods, e.g. interaction tests, and are often over-interpreted.
- Studies exploring many associations tend not to consider the increased risk of false positive findings.
- The epidemiological literature seems prone to publication bias.
- There are insufficient epidemiological publications in diseases other than cancer and cardiovascular diseases or from developing countries.
- There is a serious risk that some epidemiological publications reach misleading conclusions.

Despite the obvious merits of the GPRD the complexities of undertaking pharmacoepidemiological studies remain. This is well illustrated by two publications[11,12] that used the GPRD but reached different conclusions. The studies in question compared the incidence of venous thromboembolism among women after the UK Committee on

Safety of Medicines (now Commission on Human Medicines) advised that taking gestodene or desogestrel containing third generation oral contraceptives carried twice the risk of venous thromboembolism compared with older progestogens. One study[11] found third generation oral contraceptives were associated with twice the risk of venous thromboembolism whilst the second[12] reported results that were not consistent with a doubling of the risk of venous thromboembolism. Whatever the correct analysis the differing approaches to patient selection/exclusion and the process of dealing with confounders demonstrates the need for care by even the most experienced research worker when undertaking epidemiological studies. An analysis of 73 articles involving observational epidemiology[13] identified concerns relating to study design, size, sample selection, disease outcomes investigated, types of exposure variable, handling of confounders, methods of statistical inference, claims of effect modification, the multiplicity of outcome-exposure associations explored, and publication bias. The problems identified in this study are highlighted in Table 6.4.

Prescribing and public health

Whilst most measures of population health have shown an improvement over the past 150 years, large inequalities in health remain with the smallest improvements occurring in the health of the most disadvantaged. This is well illustrated in an analysis of data from the 865 electoral divisions in Wales.[14] Each electoral division was allocated to one of five groups according to their Townsend deprivation score. Comparison of the most deprived quintile of electoral wards to the least deprived quintile across a range of indicators of poor health or determinants of lifestyle health revealed the majority of indicators were significantly associated with deprivation as shown in Table 6.5.

With knowledge of the geographical distribution of each indicator it would appear relatively easy to map this against the prescribing of a given drug, e.g. lipid lowering agents, and determine if use was associated with one or more of a number of factors such as deprivation, consumption of a healthy diet, level of physical inactivity, number undergoing angiography or revascularisation procedures, etc. In this scenario use of proxy markers of cardiovascular morbidity to assess relative healthcare needs and comparing with the level of prescribing in a given population would appear logical. Unfortunately prescribing

TABLE 6.5 Comparison of least deprived (n=173) with most deprived (n=173) quintile of electoral wards in Wales showing those indicators significantly associated with deprivation

DOMAIN	INDICATOR	INCREASED DEPRIVATION SIGNIFICANTLY ASSOCIATED WITH INDICATOR
Lifestyle health determinant	Smoking	Yes
	Excess alcohol consumption	No
	Healthy diet	Yes
Health status	Physical inactivity	Yes
	Obesity	Yes
	Physical functioning	Yes
	Bodily pain	Yes
	General health	Yes
	Vitality	Yes
	Social functioning	Yes
	Role – emotional	Yes
	Mental health	Yes
Illness and injury	Low birth weight	Yes
	Depression and/or anxiety	Yes
	Hearing	Yes
	Eyesight	Yes
	Limiting long term illness	Yes
	Arthritis	Yes
	Back pain	Yes
	Respiratory disease	Yes
	Asthma	Yes
	Diabetes	Yes
	High blood pressure	Yes
	Heart disease	Yes
	Angina	Yes
	Heart failure	No
	Heart attack	No

DOMAIN	INDICATOR	INCREASED DEPRIVATION SIGNIFICANTLY ASSOCIATED WITH INDICATOR
	Cancer registrations	Yes
	Pedestrian injury 4–16 years reported to police	Yes
	Pedestrian injury 65+ yrs reported to police	Yes
	Pedestrian injury 5–14 yrs hospital inpatient	Yes
Use of health service	Dentist	Yes
	Family doctor	Yes
	Hospital inpatient (persons)	Yes
	CHD admission	Yes
	Angiography	Yes
	Revascularisation	Yes
	Hip replacement	No
	Knee replacement	No
	Lens replacement	Yes
Deaths	Infant mortality	Yes
	All-cause persons	Yes
	All-cause females	Yes
	All-cause males	Yes
	All cancer	Yes
	Colorectal cancer	Yes
	Lung cancer	Yes
	Breast cancer	No
	CHD	Yes
	Stroke	Yes
	Respiratory disease	Yes
	Unintentional injury	Yes
	Road traffic injury	Yes
	Unintentional fall	Yes
	Suicide	Yes

data is only routinely available at the level of the individual general medical practice and not at electoral ward level unlike the indicators of need. This can be overcome by identifying the address and post code of each patient in a given practice, calculating the proportion of individuals from each practice resident in a given ward and then allocating the prescribing profile of the practice accordingly. This has to be repeated for each practice that has patients in the electoral wards under study. Clearly there are dangers with this approach, most notably the proportional but non-weighted allocation of practice prescribing data to electoral wards that themselves could be markedly different in terms of need or deprivation.

Conclusion

In conclusion, this article has attempted to outline the scope of pharmacoepidemiological studies from the well defined methodologies that underpin a robust, scientific approach to the need for routine, pragmatic analysis of prescribing data. All methodologies discussed have limitations and it is important to be aware of these but each has its place in data analysis and an increasingly important part to play in monitoring the use of medicines in society.

References

1. Metters J. *Report of an Independent Review of access to the Yellow Card Scheme.* London: TSO; 2004.
2. Ewertz M, Mellemkjaer L, Poulsen AH, Friis S, Sorensen HT, Pedersen L, McLaughlin JK, Olsen JH. Hormone use for menopausal symptoms and risk of breast cancer. A Danish cohort study. *Br J Cancer* 2005; **92**(7): 1293–7.
3. Lindberg G, Bingefors K, Ranstam J, Råstam L, Melander A. Use of calcium channel blockers and risk of suicide: ecological findings confirmed in population based cohort study *BMJ* 1998; **316**: 741–5.
4. Lloyd DCEF, Harris CM, Roberts DJ. Specific therapeutic group age-sex weightings related prescribing units (STAR-PUs): weightings for analyzing general practices' prescribing in England. *BMJ* 1995; **311**: 991–4.
5. Avery AJ, Rodgers S, Heron T, Crombie R, Whynes D, Pringle M, Baines D, Petchey R. A prescription for improvement? An observational study to identify how general practices vary in their growth in prescribing costs. *BMJ* 2000; **321**: 276–81.
6. Prosser H, Almond S, Walley T. Influences on GPs' decision to prescribe new drugs – the importance of who says what. *Family Practice* 2003; **20**: 61–8.
7. Baxter C, Jones R, Corr L. Time trend analysis and variations in prescribing

lipid lowering drugs in general practice. *BMJ* 1998; **317**: 1134–5.

8. Scandinavian Simvastatin Survival Study Group. Randomised trial of cholesterol lowering in 4444 patients with coronary heart disease: the Scandinavian simvastatin survival study (4S). *Lancet* 1994; **344**: 1383–9.

9. Morton-Jones T, Pringle M. Explaining variations in prescribing costs across England. *BMJ* 1993; **306**: 1731–3.

10. General Practice Research Database quarterly update of bibliography: http://www.gprd.com/html/bibliography.htm (accessed January 2005).

11. Jick H, Kaye JA, Vasilakis-Scaramozza C, Jick SS. Risk of venous thromboembolism among users of third generation oral contraceptives compared with users of oral contraceptives with levonorgestrel before and after 1995: cohort and case-control analysis. *BMJ* 2000; **321**: 1190–5.

12. Farmer RDT, William TJ, Simpson EL, Nightingale AL. Effect of 1995 pill scare on rates of venous thromboembolism among women taking combined oral contraceptives: analysis of General Practice Research Database. *BMJ* 2000; **321**: 477–9.

13. Pocock SJ, Collier TJ, Dandreo KJ, de Stavola BL, Goldman MB, Kalish LA, Kasten LE, McCormack VA. Issues in the reporting of epidemiological studies: a survey of recent practice. *BMJ* 2004; **329**: 883–7.

14. National Public Health Service for Wales. Deprivation and health. Wales: NPHS, 2004. http://howis.wales.nhs.uk/sites/documents/368/Deprivationreport10Dec04.pdf (accessed January 2005).

7 Routine prescribing data

MARION BENNIE AND IAIN BISHOP

This chapter describes the data which is routinely collected within primary and secondary NHS care settings. The different sources of this data, its strengths, limitations and uses are critically reviewed. The chapter concludes with a look to the future.

Background

Nearly all patients treated within the National Health Service (NHS) receive medicines as part of their therapy. Medicines have underpinned the development of modern healthcare and it is estimated that 15–20% of the total NHS budget is spent on medicines. It is therefore critical that we have systems to understand how we are using medicines in the NHS and ultimately what health gain is achieved. This chapter will examine primary care and hospital prescribing; outline the current tools available, their uses, benefits and limitations and end with a view to the future.

Primary care prescribing information

Prescribing information can come in a number of different forms, depending on the source of the information, the processing authority, and the format in which it is presented. This chapter aims to describe the array of prescribing information available and its potential uses. However, before progressing any further it is important to make the distinction between prescribing information and prescribing statistics.

Prescribing statistics

Prescribing statistics are published on behalf of each of the home countries' parliaments and are collated figures covering the country as a total. They provide information broken down by cost and volume for each *British National Formulary* (BNF) chapter. Sites providing prescribing statistics are listed below.

- http://www.publications.doh.gov.uk/prescriptionstatistics/
- http://www.isdscotland.org/isd/info3.jsp?pContentID=1041&p_applic=CCC&p_service=Content.show&
- http://www.wales.nhs.uk/sites3/page.cfm?orgid=428&pid=13533
- http://www.centralservicesagency.com/display/statistics

Prescribing information

Prescribing information could be described as prescribing statistics provided at a more detailed level, sufficient to analyse the prescribing patterns of individual prescribers, or groups of prescribers. It can also be provided in small enough aliquots, e.g. monthly, to provide analyses of change over time as well as comparisons in single time periods. It is the availability and uses of this type of prescribing information that form the focus of this chapter. It is important to note at this point that health services have responsibilities under both the Freedom of Information Act and the Data Protection Act that informs data access for different users.

Data sources

The data which enables the production of primary care prescribing information is generated as a by-product of the processing of prescriptions, for the purpose of reimbursing the costs of drugs which have been dispensed by community pharmacists, dispensing doctors and appliance suppliers. These prescriptions will have been written by any of the currently acceptable prescriber types, e.g. general practitioner (GP), nurse prescriber, community pharmacist prescriber (*see also* Chapter 10); or by authorised secondary care prescribers on specific prescription forms, which can be dispensed in the community, e.g. HBP prescriptions in Scotland.

The monthly processing and pricing of prescriptions is carried out by the relevant processing body as listed below.

- England: Prescription Pricing Division (PPD) (http://www.ppa. org.uk/ppa/ppa_main.htm)
- Wales: Prescribing Services Unit, Health Solutions Wales (http:// www.wales.nhs.uk/sites3/page.cfm?orgid=166&pid=3997)
- Scotland: Practitioner Services Division, NHS National Services Scotland (http://www.psd.scot.nhs.uk/)
- North Ireland: (http://www.centralservicesagency.com/display/ pharmaceuticalservices)

Following processing, data is passed to other departments within each country's processing body to map to the prescriber codes necessary to create prescriber based information from the prescription based data.

This data is then made available at different levels to different user groups, e.g. prescribing advisers to monitor the clinical and cost effectiveness of prescribing for a geographical area; practitioners providing services to support clinical audit; and finance and health authorities to enable planning and performance management.

England (PACT/ePACT)

PACT (prescribing analysis and cost) data is collated and made available in a series of reports from the PPA. The reports inform general practices and prescribers which drugs and appliances have been prescribed, and their expenditure for a given period. Reports consist of aggregated information.

ePACT.net is an application that allows authorised users to view and analyse PACT data from the PPA. More information on the use of ePACT is available from http://www.ppa.org.uk/news/help/epact. net/pcg/usgLoggingon.htm

Scotland (SPA/PRISMS)

SPA (Scottish Prescribing Analysis) is made available to all general practices and prescribers. SPA is available at two levels:
- SPA Level 1, sent automatically to GPs, is a breakdown of total costs and number of items dispensed for major therapeutic categories compared against averages for the practice, NHS board, and Scotland
- SPA Level 2, originally produced on request for GPs, practice or NHS board shows all items dispensed in a three-month period.

PRISMS (PRescribing Information SysteM for Scotland) is a web-based application, giving access to prescribing information for all prescriptions dispensed in the community for the past five years.

The information is held centrally and is updated monthly. This data can be interrogated to provide reports at practice level and aggregate data to a Scotland level. Work is currently ongoing to make SPA level 1 and 2 data available via PRISMS. More information about PRISMS is only available via an NHSnet connection at the following URL: www.primsmsweb.scot.nhs.uk/.

Wales (CASPA)

CASPA (Comparative Analysis System for Prescribing Audit) is a desktop prescribing analysis system provided by Health Solutions Wales.

Northern Ireland (COMPASS)

COMPASS is a prescribing information system developed to provide GPs with feedback on their prescribing (COMPASS Prescribing Report). This is supplemented with evidence-based advice on the use of medicines which is provided to GPs and pharmacists.

In exploring further the range of prescribing information available the assumption has been made that the Wales and Northern Ireland systems have similar functionality to ePACT or PRISMS.

Prescribing measures

Before considering the benefits and limitations of using prescribing information, it is important to consider the prescribing measures generated by prescribing information systems. This is important because there are a number of different measures that can be used to analyse prescribing. Using an inappropriate measure may provide a view of the data that is completely spurious. Therefore understanding these measures and their appropriate use is essential to efficient and effective provision of prescribing information. Examples with explanatory comment are provided throughout this section to aid understanding.

Traditional prescribing measures
Quantity

Common physical units, e.g. grams, litres, number of tablets, and number of items are used to quantify drug usage. These units should be applied only when the use of one drug, or of specific products, is being evaluated. Problems arise when it is used in the context of utilisation of whole drug groups. If usage is given in terms of grams of active ingredients, drugs with low potency will have a larger fraction of the total than drugs with high potency. Counting numbers of tablets also has disadvantages because strengths of tablets vary. The result is that low strength preparations contribute relatively more than high strength preparations. In addition, short-acting products will contribute more than long-acting preparations.

There are some instances where number of items does not give a good indication of total use unless total amount of drug per item is also considered. Counting items is of more value in measuring the frequency of prescribing and this is relevant to treatments given largely, or entirely, as courses, e.g. antibiotics and immunisations. Other factors can confound these measures, such as the size of the practice population, i.e. a large practice is likely to prescribe more in absolute terms than a small one. It is therefore sometimes better for comparative purposes to refer to items per 1000 patients. This method and other similar measures are described in more detail later.

Expenditure
There are two ways of expressing expenditure related to prescribing. The various countries name these differently, which is often confusing.

List price
The list price is the basic price of a drug, i.e. the price listed in the *Drug Tariff* or the *Monthly Index of Medical Specialities* (MIMS). List price is used in PACT reports, PRISMS and other analyses reflecting the prescribing performance of GPs and health authorities. The list price is known as gross ingredient cost (GIC) in Scotland and net ingredient cost (NIC) in England.

Reimbursement price
Reimbursement price is closer to the true price paid by the NHS. Community pharmacists are reimbursed for prescriptions they have dispensed on the basis of the list price less the discount that they are assumed to have received from their suppliers. This is known as net ingredient cost (NIC) in Scotland and 'actual cost' in England.

When prescribing is analysed it is more appropriate to use the list price as it allows accurate comparisons between practices. However, from a financial perspective, the NHS needs to know the reimbursement price. In many cases prescribing advisers will project in terms of list price and accountants will convert these figures to reimbursement price.

For the purposes of clarity all examples will use the Scottish terms GIC (list price) and NIC (reimbursement price). Some examples to illustrate this are shown below. All examples use the prescribing of a group of drugs known as statins for the same group of practices for the same time period.

Figure 7.1 shows cost and volume for statin prescribing over a three month period for a random selection of GP practices. The variance in both volume and cost between practices is significant. This may be due in part to practice population effects. Additionally, the pattern of expenditure does not fully match the volume pattern. This may be the effect of the repeat prescription cycle length and/ or specific drug choices in each practice and/or levels of generic prescribing. With this number of potential variables affecting the information, further refining of the data is needed to provide more meaningful comparisons.

Figure 7.2 provides an insight into whether the quantity prescribed has an effect on the understanding of the data. The quantity pattern

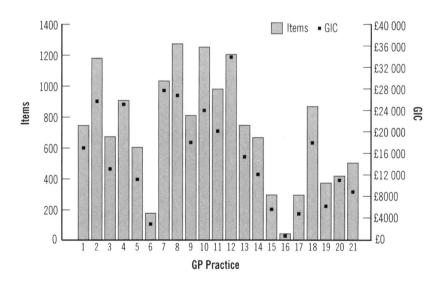

FIGURE 7.1 Statin prescribing for a three-month period for a group of GP practices

in Figure 7.2 is very similar to the cost pattern in Figure 7.1. However, if practices 7 and 12 are looked at in detail it can be seen that the quantities are relatively higher than the number of items, suggesting larger quantities per prescription being issued.

To enhance clarity and flexibility in analysis it is possible to derive further measures from the data. These fall into two main categories: prescription derived measures, and population derived measures. Some of these measures are specific to particular prescribing information systems and may not all be available in any one system.

Prescription derived measures
Cost per item
The cost per item measure is a simple division of the costs by the number of items. This can be a helpful measure in standardising data with regards to the number of prescriptions written thereby minimising the effect of practice population size.

Figure 7.3 uses the same practices as Figures 7.1 and 7.2 and shows both the number of items prescribed along with the cost per item for statins. The patterns for both GIC and quantity in Figures 7.1 and 7.2 differ completely from the pattern for GIC/item in Figure 7.3.

In Figure 7.2 it was shown that two practices (7 and 12) were prescribing larger quantities than the other practices. However, we

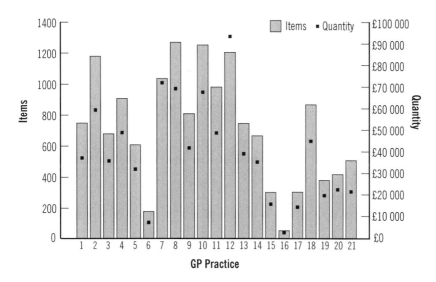

FIGURE 7.2 Statin prescribing for a three-month period for a group of GP practices

can see that there are four practices whose GIC/item is higher than the rest. These are practices 4, 7, 12, and 20. This suggests that whilst the quantities prescribed by practices 7 and 12 may be influencing their high GIC/item, this cannot explain the high GIC/item for practice 4 and 20. In this case the high GIC/item may be a function of three possible factors:

- higher strengths being prescribed
- differences in product choice
- high brand, low generic prescribing.

To achieve further clarity, the questions asked and the data retrieved need to be refined.

Average quantity per item

This measure is derived by dividing the total quantity prescribed by the total number of items prescribed, and can be used to confirm the assumptions in Figure 7.2.

Defined daily doses

Defined daily doses (DDDs) are a World Health Organization (WHO) statistical measure of drug consumption. DDDs are used to standardise the comparative usage of various drugs. They are a

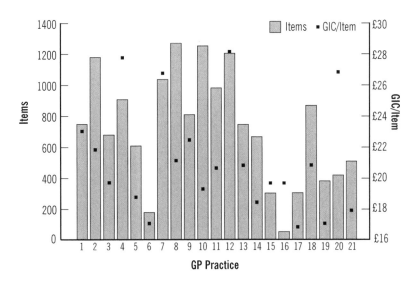

FIGURE 7.3 Statin prescribing for a three-month period for a group of GP practices

function of strength and quantity, and the basic definition of the unit given by the WHO is: 'The DDD is the assumed average maintenance dose per day for a drug used for its main indication in adults.'

It should be emphasised that the DDD is a unit of measurement and does not necessarily reflect the recommended or prescribed daily dose. Doses for individual patients and patient groups will often differ from the DDD and will necessarily have to be based on individual characteristics (e.g. age and weight) and pharmacokinetic considerations. The DDD is nearly always a compromise based on a review of the available information including the dosages used in various countries when this information is available. The DDD is sometimes a dose that is rarely if ever prescribed, because it is an average of two or more commonly used dosage regimes.

Drug consumption data presented as DDDs only gives a rough estimate of consumption and not an exact picture of actual use. DDDs provide a fixed unit of measurement independent of price and formulation enabling the researcher to assess trends in drug consumption and to perform comparisons between population groups.

DDDs are not established for topical preparations, sera, vaccines, antineoplastic agents, allergen extracts, general and local anaesthetics, nor are they available for combination products.

The formula for calculating DDDs is as follows:

$$\text{Drug Usage (DDDs)} = \left(\frac{\text{Items issued} \times \text{Amount of Drug per item}}{\text{WHO DDD Measure}} \right)$$

For example, paracetamol has a WHO DDD of 3g. If a patient is issued with a prescription for 84 × paracetamol 500mg tablets, the prescription could be said to contain 14 DDDs of paracetamol – calculated as 1 item containing 42g (84 × 0.5g), divided by 3g.

For more information on DDDs, visit the website http://www.whocc.no/atcddd/ and *see also* Chapter 6.

DDDs per item

This can be considered to be similar to average quantity per item. It standardises the data effect of total volumes (both items and quantity) and population sizes. It can be used to confirm larger quantities and/or higher strengths per prescription. The effect of using this measure is shown in Figure 7.4.

In Figure 7.4 practices 4 and 20 show high GIC/DDD, but practices 7 and 12 do not. This does suggest, but does not completely confirm, that practices 4 and 20 tend to prescribe statins that have a higher cost per DDD, i.e. newer preparations or proprietary brands rather

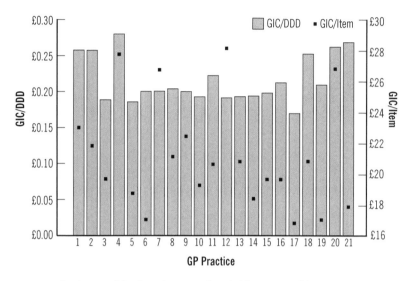

FIGURE 7.4 Statin prescribing for a three-month period for a group of GP practices

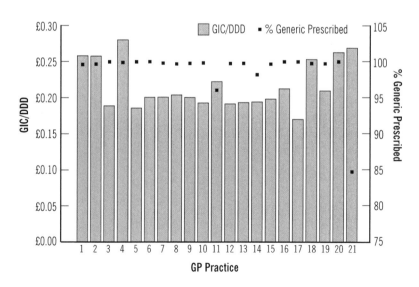

FIGURE 7.5 Statin prescribing for a three-month period for a group of GP practices

than generic versions of established medicines. Querying generic prescribing rates might further clarify this point.

Generic prescribing rates

Generic prescribing rates for the same group of drugs are shown in Figure 7.5. However, this fails to illustrate any real differences in generic prescribing rates between practices 4, 7, 12 and 20. The only practices with relatively low generic prescribing rates are practices 11 and 21. This does support the hypothesis that practice 4 and 20 may prescribe generically in general, but preferred to use a statin for which there is no generic product available, such as a more recently marketed drug entity, only available as a branded product.

Average daily quantity

DDDs have been based on international prescribing habits. Work done by the Prescribing Support Unit (PSU) (http://www.ic.nhs.uk/our-services/prescribing-support) demonstrated that prescribing by GPs in England could differ from the international standard. To allow comparison of prescribing within England there was a need to have a system that more accurately reflected English GPs' prescribing. The result was the development of average daily quantities (ADQs) by an expert group convened by the PSU.

ADQs are not recommended doses but are analytical units produced in order to compare more accurately the prescribing activity of primary care practitioners in England. More information on ADQs is also mentioned in Chapter 6. http://www.ppa.org.uk/news/help/toolkit/pre_meas.htm#prescribed%20daily%20dosen

Population derived measures

The volume and cost of prescribing are influenced by the demography and morbidity of the population served, e.g. on average, elderly patients have a greater need for medicines than younger adult patients. These should, therefore, wherever possible and appropriate, be taken into account when comparing data either between GP practices or at higher organisational levels.

Unweighted patients

The population, i.e. number of patients for a given practice, area, health authority or NHS board is their unweighted patient population. It is unweighted in that the population figure is unadulterated by

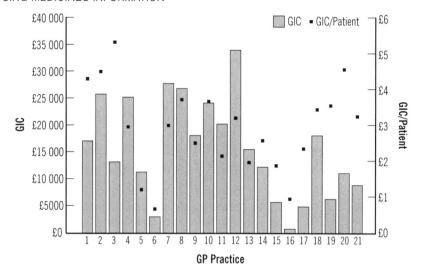

FIGURE 7.6 Statin prescribing for a three-month period for a group of GP practices

additional demographic and morbidity factors which could affect the uptake and use of medicines, e.g. age, gender, deprivation, chronic illnesses, and thus confound comparisons between groups.

Cost per patient

This measure is similar to cost per item, but uses the practice population as the denominator of the measure. This measure adjusts for the effects of population size and prescription volume.

Figure 7.6 details the differences between overall expenditure (GIC) and cost per patient (GIC/Patient). It is apparent that high overall GIC does not necessary relate to high GIC/Patient.

Items per 1000 patients

This is calculated by dividing the total items by the practice population, then multiplying by 1000. This is shown in Figure 7.7.

By using both the GIC/Patient (Figure 7.6) and Items/1000 Patients (Figure 7.7) we can separate out practices which could truly be considered 'High cost/High volume' for further analysis. In this example, practices 3 and 20 would require further investigation.

Weighted patients

Adding a weighting to a patient population attempts to recalculate an

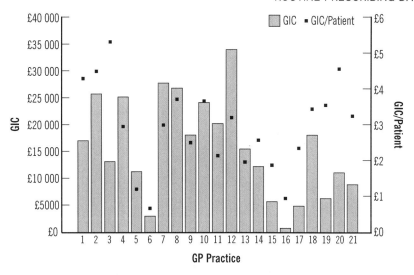

FIGURE 7.7 Statin prescribing for a three-month period for a group of GP practices

assumed higher or lower medicines usage as a result of demographic and morbidity factors within the population. It does this by means of inflating or deflating the population figure, e.g. if a particular practice has a population of 3000, but if the patients are particularly elderly or live in a deprived area, the weighted population of the practice could be 4000. There have been many different approaches to developing weighting formulae, some of which are described below, none of which are considered a gold standard throughout the UK.

The Arbuthnott Formula

In Scotland, the Arbuthnott Formula is used as a weighting measure for populations. The formula takes account of the population in the NHS board area, the age of the population, gender, level of deprivation and the proportion of population living in remote and rural areas. More information on the Arbuthnott Formula is available here: http://www.scotland.gov.uk/Publications/2005/10/19160721/07218

Figure 7.8 shows the differences between practices using unweighted and weighted populations.

ASTRO-PU

ASTRO-PUs (age sex temporary resident originated prescribing units)

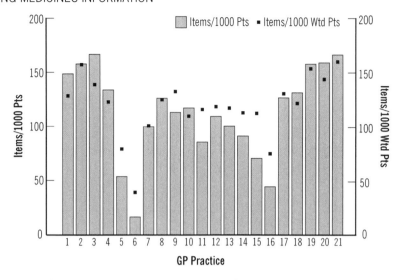

FIGURE 7.8 Statin prescribing for a three-month period for a group of GP practices

were derived by the Prescribing Research Unit (PRU) in 1993. Detailed information on their construction and use is available at http://www. ic.nhs.uk/our-services/prescribing-support-unit/measures/astro-pus. *See also* Chapter 6.

STAR-PU

STAR-PUs (specific therapeutic age-sex related prescribing units) were derived in 1995. Detailed information on their use is available at http:// www.ic.nhs.uk/our-services/prescribing-support/measures/ star-pus. *See also* Chapter 6.

Application of ASTRO-PUs and STAR-PUs would be similar in principle to the illustration using Arbuthnott (Figure 7.8) but would differ in exact details of the effect.

Benefits of prescribing information

The benefits of correctly analysed and used prescribing information are many. However, prescribing information must be seen as a means of adding richness to the data available. It can act as a catalyst for discussion by using it to formulate more reasoned and intelligent questions. It is only when prescribing activity is combined with an understanding of the underlying clinical evidence and used as part of discussions and debates with prescribers regarding their clinical use of medicines that a fuller level of knowledge can begin to emerge.

The following include examples of areas in which prescribing information can be beneficial. They are exemplars and are not intended to be exhaustive.

Planning

Prescribing information can be used to identify both clinical and financial risks to organisations and policymakers to support clinical service development and budget allocation.

Budget allocation

Budget allocation can be approached using regression analysis of the prescribing cost trends, integrated with other elements that can affect the potential expenditure over a projected period, e.g.

- drugs losing patent protection (exclusivity of the manufacturer for the market for a defined period) and lower cost generic equivalents becoming available
- entry of new drugs into the marketplace
- new clinical evidence that could increase or decrease the use of a medicine or group of medicines.

Financial risk management

Changing prescribing which deviates from predictions can create financial risk for an organisation. Close monitoring of medicines usage, even with the natural delay in prescribing information (usually about three months), can support contingency planning.

Clinical and cost effectiveness use of medicines

Monitoring of new drug uptake is of particular importance to understand how these medicines are being used in general practice compared to the clinical trial setting. This is of specific importance for drugs reviewed by National Institute for Health and Clinical Excellence (NICE) and the Scottish Medicines Consortium (SMC). In addition, the ability to review changes in prescribing behaviour following the publication of landmark trials is useful.

Exception reporting

As can be seen from the examples given there is the potential to retrieve vast quantities of data and eventually suffer from 'paralysis by analysis', i.e. having so much data that you become overwhelmed and unable to find a logical way forward. To prevent this situation from occurring, there are occasions where exception reporting should be used. In these situations identification of changes outside the norm are worthy of further investigation. This is not to say that higher or lower than average use is good or bad, but that it is different, and until a clinical context is placed on the prescribing activity then the activity needs to be questioned.

Changing service models

Monitoring the impact of new services or contracts, e.g. in the new General Medical Services (GMS) contract, a number of specific drugs and groups of drugs are linked explicitly or implicitly to the Quality and Outcomes Framework (QOF). The changes in use of these medicines can be monitored over time by practice to gauge the effects of the new contract on clinical activity and expenditure, and can often identify contrasting activity by neighbouring practices, e.g. one practice opting for the most potent statin available in order to reach the highest possible threshold and earn the higher number of QOF points in that section regardless of the effect on prescribing expenditure, whilst another practice selecting the most cost effective generic product first line and only moving onto another, more potent (and more expensive) statin when patients fail to reach the appropriate cholesterol target.

Changing prescribers' prescribing activity

One of the most effective ways of influencing change is showing prescribers comparisons of themselves against their peers. This is often best carried out in the form of a graph showing the particular practice in the context of a group of practices. Following agreement with practices regarding courses of action, positive feedback using prescribing information throughout the process of change can help to maintain the momentum of something that can take considerable time and effort to change.

Prescribing indicators

Providing comparisons is extremely useful, especially if a prescribing indicator for a particular clinical activity can be developed. The benefit here is that the measurement can be standardised. For example, one current public health message is that individuals should not exceed 6g per day of salt intake. However, if patients are prescribed effervescent formulations of paracetamol or co-codamol and take eight tablets per day, they will receive 8.8g of salt per day in addition to any dietary intake. Therefore a prescribing indicator showing effervescent formulations of these products as a percentage of all similar thera-peutic, but non-effervescent, formulations can inform measures to reduce the inappropriate use of these formulations. The indicator can be calculated using measures of 'quantity' (probably more accurate) or 'items' (probably less accurate), but the important point is that it has to be measured and calculated consistently. Prescribing indica-tors can be used incorrectly; therefore, it is important to remember that their use may indicate something unusual or different from the norm, but this may not necessarily be good or bad. A clinical context must always be sought.

Formulary compliance

Providing comparisons of a number of practices' compliance with either locally or nationally produced formularies is another useful tool. It should be noted, however, that unless the formulary is totally inclusive of all available products, then compliance will always be lower than 100%. In many instances a reasonable level of compliance with a locally based formulary is likely to be in the range of 70–90%.

Limitations of prescribing information

Whilst there are many benefits of using appropriately analysed prescribing information, there are also limitations in its use. These must always be taken into account when reviewing prescribing information. Some of the key issues are discussed below.

Data accuracy

The most fundamental limiting factor is the accuracy of the base data used to generate prescribing information. Without an understanding of the base data accuracy, confidence in the information provided via prescribing information systems can be eroded.

Prescription handling within practices

The first level of data inaccuracy lies within practices themselves. The process in place within the practice for dealing with repeat prescriptions (approximately 80% of the total prescription volume) will determine accuracy, or lack of it, at prescriber level. Most clinical systems have the facility within them to either print the cipher (code) of the GP who will sign the prescription, or the cipher of the GP with whom the patient is registered. If the latter option is chosen, the prescribing is attributed to the GP the patient is registered with. This may not be the GP the patient regularly sees, or who initiated the therapy. Therefore care must be taken when attempting to analyse data at individual prescriber level as inaccuracy in the data may be high.

Processing

Once prescriptions have been dispensed they are returned by the community pharmacy to be processed for payment. This processing inevitably has a level of error that can add to data inaccuracy. Most processing systems operate at accuracy rates of about 99%, which appears high, but when converted to actual prescriptions, it means that over the whole of the UK some 600,000–700,000 prescriptions are potentially incorrectly processed each month.

Patient characteristics

Since prescribing information is generated from prescriptions dispensed, there is currently no link to the GP clinical system or the community pharmacy patient medication record, and therefore no current linkage to patient identifiable data.

Demographics

There is no information available within prescribing information systems currently which indicates the socioeconomic class of the patient, or the rurality of their abode. However, work in Scotland is progressing to promote the use and capture of the Community Health Index (CHI) from primary care prescriptions which will enable age, gender and post code to be established for individual patients enabling prescribing to be assigned to the patient's residence rather than the general practice providing services.

Morbidity

There is currently no indication on prescriptions as to the clinical reason for the prescription being written. There is also no indication of whether this is initiation of new therapy or continuation therapy.

Such information would support pharmacoepidemiology and pharmacovigilance (*see* Chapters 6 and 9).

Hospital prescribing information

In comparison to primary care there is currently a paucity of hospital prescribing information available at a national level. This is a consequence of a number of factors including:

- numerous different hospital medicine stock control systems currently in place in NHS hospitals across the UK
- no standardisation of medicine dictionaries within and across these systems
- until recently, few drivers to encourage benchmarking across comparable hospitals in respect to medicines utilisation
- greater focus on primary care prescribing in part due to higher expenditure in comparison to hospital prescribing, i.e. approximately 90% primary care and 10% secondary care.

It should, however, be recognised that locally hospitals have had a long history of using information on medicines utilisation at a clinical level to support evidence-based medicine. This grew from the original hospital based formulary management system into full clinical pharmacy services to support patient care. Formulary management provides a process that enables clinicians to agree upon a selected number of medicines for routine use within the clinical settings to:

- support evidence-based practice
- enable familiarity with a range of medicines to minimise medication errors with a particular focus on supporting new prescribers
- facilitate communication across different specialities
- support the management of the medicines distribution system
- feedback on the usage of medicines within defined clinical areas.

These developments in hospital prescribing information have supported the development of the current primary care systems available nationally. It is now time to reflect on the experience with national primary care prescribing information to inform the building of secondary care systems to meet the information needs of clinicians, planners, policymakers and the public in the future.

Data sources

Work continues across the UK to assist in providing an interim solution to the data deficit in hospital prescribing information. The long term vision is for hospital prescribing information to be a by-product of the introduction of electronic prescribing and administration systems which will require the use of a standardised medicines dictionary. This is part of the wider single patient record initiative within the NHS.

The following is an outline of work ongoing in England and developmental work in Scotland to provide interim data on hospital prescribing.

England

England currently has no central collation of medicines used and issued in NHS hospitals. However, the NHS Health and Social Care Information Centre, a special health authority, has published in 2005 its first bulletin on hospital prescribing, generated from the Hospital Pharmacy Audit Index (HPAI). This data source is produced by IMS Health, a commercial company. IMS Health collects and collates all information on medicines issued from hospital pharmacy depart-ments covering 97% of NHS hospitals in England. This first bulletin provides overall costs of medicines by health authority combining primary and secondary care data and also seeks to look at specific therapeutic areas and specific drugs, approved through NICE. (http://www.ic.nhs.uk/statistics-and-data-collections/primary-care/prescribing/hospital-prescribing-2004--england)

Information on hospital outpatient prescribing (FP10) is routinely collated through ePACT and designated hospital ePACT data (www.ppa.org.uk). Hospital outpatient prescribing varies across the UK dependent upon the model of health service delivery, e.g. outpatient prescriptions dispensed through community pharmacies in Scotland is minimal in comparison with England.

Scotland

Scotland like England has no central collation of hospital medicines usage. However, work has commenced through NHS National Services Scotland, a special health board, to explore the building of a national hospital database to enable submission of data from all hospital pharmacy departments in Scotland. This programme of work is linked to and will help to inform the national programme for the introduction of hospital electronic prescribing and medicines administration (HEPMA), a by-product of which will be medicines utilisation data. This database will initially provide high level expenditure data by *BNF* category at hospital, health board, regional and national levels. With time this will extend to provide detailed medicines utilisation data on specific clinical areas and specific drugs including key drugs recommended for use by the Scottish Medicines Consortium (SMC). The SMC provides single technology assessments near to or at the point of launch for all new medicines and major new indications for the NHS in Scotland.

Prescribing measures

As outlined previously there are a number of prescribing measures that can be used to present prescribing information. The traditional measures of volume and expenditure remain the mainstay of current data, the most predominant of these being total expenditure, generally assimilated to *BNF* categories.

Application of DDDs to hospital prescribing data is a growing area of development to assist in standardisation of data by taking into account the volume and strength of the medicine. For example: the ability to summate the total amount of antibiotic prescribed across primary and secondary care for a geographical area can support the understanding of the exposure of the population and potential relationship to the generation of antimicrobial resistance.

Population-derived measures in the context of hospital prescribing are restricted at present by the established data capture systems which focus on hospital activity rather than the population demographics and characteristics. The most frequently used generic measures are:

- occupied bed days
- admissions, e.g. Scottish Morbidity Records (SMR) – admissions and referral rates by clinical speciality, admissions by diagnostic category and operative procedures; English hospital episodes statistics
- consultant episodes.

The major limitation of these measures with respect to prescribing data is the inherent variability in our hospital populations due to the development of different service delivery models and clinical specialities which impact significantly on the interpretation of such prescribing information. For example, a large tertiary referral centre is likely to have a different population, prescribing and service delivery profile than a local district general hospital. In such situations the need for careful benchmarking is critical and the risk of misinterpretation is potentially higher than for a general practice population. Access to hospital activity data is through the prescribing statistics websites identified at the start of this chapter.

Future developments in prescribing information

The future use of prescribing information is dependent on ensuring that prescribing data, both primary and secondary care, is routinely captured as a by-product of clinical care and not a separate activity either to enable payment to contractors/clinicians for services undertaken or by hospitals to demonstrate performance. Linkage directly to patient care and integration within the single patient record system will support appropriate record linkage of prescribing to clinical condition and clinical outcome, a much better information stream on which to support continuous quality improvement.

A number of areas require research and development if we are to maximise the rich data streams to evolve from the single patient record.

- How do we best present information to support clinicians to continuously improve prescribing given the extended ability to link prescribing to patient characteristics and clinical conditions?
- How do we better support routine pharmacovigilance and generation of early warning signals for potentially unknown adverse effects to medicines?
- How do we utilise the routine capture of population data to establish the clinical effectiveness of medicines outwith strict clinical trial settings?
- How do we convert these richer datasets into knowledge to support efficient and effective policymaking, service planning and performance management?

Conclusion

Primary care prescribing information can be extremely useful in the forecasting of medicines usage and identification of clinical and financial risks. It can be an extremely good catalyst for change when correctly contextualised, but there remain some potentially confounding limitations to the data and how it relates to patients in the clinical setting. It is therefore vitally important that when using prescribing information, the data is contextualised as accurately as possible including the limitations of the data if it is to be optimally used.

However, hospital prescribing data is still underutilised, at a national level, due to practical and logistical reasons reflecting the historical development of the systems at individual sites rather than as a centrally co-ordinated and supported programme.

In summary, there have been considerable developments in pre-scribing information in the last 10–15 years but the next 10–15 years should see further major advancements in this field if information management and technology can be effectively harnessed in the field of healthcare delivery. Medicines will remain a driving force in the advancement and delivery of healthcare. It is therefore critical that we have the systems and the intelligence to use the data generated through the application of such technology within the NHS to understand the health gain achieved through such investment of public monies.

8 Health economic uses of drug data

STEPHEN CHAPMAN

This chapter describes the changing emphasis on cost and cost effectiveness of medicines which has developed in parallel with their increasing use, and implications for NHS budgets. It illustrates how routine data can be used both to identify and chart savings which the NHS can achieve by considered use of therapeutic equivalents within drug classes. Some of the limitations in using such high level anonymised data, which cannot be linked to individual patients needs and outcomes, are also highlighted.

From willow trees to aspirin

Back in 490 BC, at what could be considered to be the dawn of modern medicine, Hippocrates was not unduly bothered by the cost of his pharmaceutical interventions. He stripped the bark from willow trees, boiled it up and made a mild infusion of what we now know to be salicylic acid. Clinical risks and benefits may well have been considered, but are not recorded. The solution was a reasonable analgesic and anti-febrile agent but we have no information on whether or not possible gastro-intestinal bleeds manifested. Be that as it may, willow trees grew freely and water was freely available, as was the source of heat to boil the water.

The manufacture and formulation of medicines developed in much the same way over the centuries: the therapeutic properties of more plants were investigated and were variously turned into solutions, powders, pills, suspensions, infusions and poultices. Those with the skills to identify their correct 'materia medica' and formulate them appropriately charged for both their services as apothecaries and for the finished product. Throughout this time the principle of 'caveat emptor', that is 'buyer beware', operated. The apothecaries and herbalists made whatever claim they wanted for the infusions or solutions they supplied and it was up to the potential patient to decide whether the investment of their money was a reasonable risk to take to alleviate their suffering.

Things started to change at the very end of the 19th century. A chemist named Felix Hoffman, working at Bayer in Germany, chemically synthesised a stable form of acetalsalicylic acid as a powder and used it to relieve his father's rheumatism. Bayer distributed what became known as aspirin powder worldwide from 1899, thus becoming the first major pharmaceutical company. By 1900, aspirin was available as water soluble tablets, and was the first medication to be sold in this form. At about the same time, Alexander Fleming was exploring the use of various products to try to lyse bacterial cells and by chance identified the antibiotic properties of the fungus penicillium. Subsequently penicillin became known as the first antibiotic. Initially it was only used to treat soldiers during the First World War, but after a high profile fire at a Boston club, when the company Merck used a large supply of penicillin to treat the patients at Massachusetts General Hospital, national headlines led to widespread public awareness of the powers of antibiotics.

At this point, 'caveat emptor' still existed and the drugs could be bought and sold as commodities by the public. But, these newly developed, mass produced drugs started to raise previously unexplored ethical dilemmas; it was possible to make drugs on a large scale that could treat debilitating conditions, and in the case of antibiotics, save life, but they were not affordable to all.

Flawed assumptions and practical realities

In the UK, in the immediate post-Second World War period, there was a need for a substantive workforce for the manufacturing industry, but an employment shortage existed. The major morbidities at the time were acute illnesses such as tuberculosis and polio. The National Health Service was thus developed to make medical care free at the point of access, and medicines available on prescription at no fee, or a nominal low fee, irrespective of the cost of the drug. It was assumed that, as a consequence, the workforce would be fit to return to work more quickly, thus generating more income and taxes. It was expected that the system would pay for itself. The other change this precipitated was the principle of the doctor acting as the patient's agent in determining access to healthcare and medicines. This produced a paradigm shift in responsibility – it was no longer the patient themselves who decided on the balance of cost and effectiveness of the desired drug, but the prescriber acting on their behalf.

As the Health Service became more established and a generation passed, free access to doctors and prescriptions for medicines became the norm. Thus both doctors and their patients had come to expect that in the majority of cases a consultation with a GP would end with a prescription for medicine. Indeed this 'pill for every ill' culture became so ingrained in society that doctors began to feel they could not end a consultation and thus relieve time pressure on surgeries, without issuing a prescription. Patients, in some cases, felt they were getting less than optimal treatment if they didn't receive a prescription for medication when they went for their appointment.

This situation is most apparent, and oft quoted by doctors and patients alike, when prescriptions for antibiotics were considered. Doctors under time pressure felt the issue of a cheap antibiotic prescription would help them ease the patient out of the surgery and allow them onto their next consultation, and subsequently patients with coughs and colds, which may have been of viral origin, had come to expect that they should be treated with an antibiotic 'just in case'. The public health implications of mass prescribing of antibiotics in this way, and the development of antibiotic resistance, were in fact highlighted in the early days by Alexander Fleming. But as long as new antibiotics continued to come on the market, these warnings were by and large ignored, and new and more powerful agents appeared to replace those that were becoming ineffective. It was only towards the end of the 20th century that prescribers and policymakers realised that this had to stop. The first step was for prescribers to be cognisant of the quantity and cost of the medicines they prescribed.

Putting to one side the clinical implications, it was obvious that cost was not a major consideration when doctors were issuing high volumes of prescriptions. This rather artificial distancing from the financial pressures of medicines ceased abruptly in the 1990s with the advent of the then Conservative Government's policy of 'purchase/provider split'. This policy, along with general practice fundholding, meant that doctors were now costing out services they were commissioning from the hospitals. In addition, they were being given information on the cost of their prescribing, for which, in the case of fundholders, they were totally financially responsible. Any savings made from the drugs budget by not prescribing, or prescribing cheaper equivalent medicines, were retained by the practice, and could be re-invested for improving patient healthcare. For fundholders and non-fundholders alike, though, this presented a problem. What data could be usefully employed to help them optimise their prescribing?

Data rich and information poor?

The routine key dataset currently commonly available to general practice prescribers is PACT data (*see also* Chapter 7). PACT data is available at practice, primary care trust, strategic health authority and national level. Originally the data comprised paper reports but are now available electronically via epact.net. Trend data shows the rate of increase in either the cost or volume of a particular class or group of drugs. PACT can also be used for comparative data at practice or PCT level. This data can be used for crude and pragmatic health economic analysis; that is, *cost minimisation*. Put simply, when two agents or interventions can be shown to have identical outcomes then the cheaper agent of the two is selected. If a practice, or PCT, wants to reduce the rate of rise to minimise their costs, they can use PACT data as a guide towards cost minimisation. For instance, Figure 8.1 shows the trends for cardiovascular drugs, including statin prescribing, of a PCT. Figure 8.2 shows the relative costs for a comparative group of PCTs.

The most basic form of cost minimisation, and most commonly applied, is the use of generic medicines rather than brands. As the generic manufacturer has not had to invest in R&D costs, and recover the overheads, they can afford to price the medicine at the cost of its manufacture, plus profit margin, which is significantly lower than the cost of the brand leader. The majority of prescribers now prescribe medicines by their generic name routinely, so this switch often takes place by default as soon as the medicine is out of patent. In those instances when it does not take place by default, it is a relatively simple job on most GPs' software to substitute a generic product for its branded equivalent by overtyping or pressing the 'G' button which does it automatically. Data such as that in Figure 8.2 helps show the potential for savings from generic switches.

Figure 8.2 also illustrates how data can be used for more sophisticated economic modelling by looking at the cost implications of switching between agents. This is a form of *cost-effectiveness analysis*.

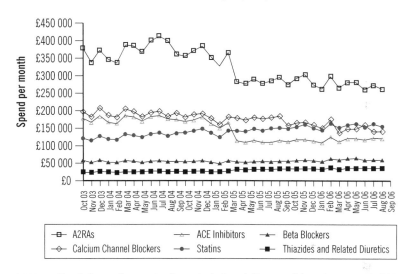

FIGURE 8.1 Trends for cardiovascular drugs, including statin prescribing, of an example PCT

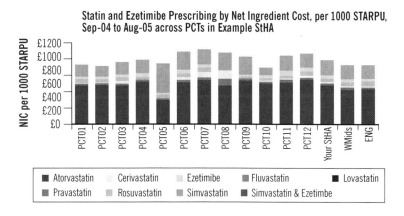

FIGURE 8.2 Relative costs for a comparative group of PCTs

In cost-effective analysis, the cost of treatment is compared with the expected outcome measured in natural units, in this case reduction in cholesterol. The costs of the intervention per unit of clinical outcome are compared. If one assumes that the majority of the statins in Figure 8.2 will reduce cholesterol, and that the majority of patients will respond to simvastatin, it is reasonable to suggest that if all new patients are started on generic simvastatin cost savings will result. In a typical PCT, this can be modelled as shown in Table 8.1.

TABLE 8.1 Modelled savings generated by initiating new patients on generic simvastatin 40mg

| YEAR | SAVINGS FROM PRESCRIBING NEW STATIN DDDS AS SIMVASTATIN 40MG | | | |
	10% NEW AS SIMVASTATIN 40MG	25% NEW AS SIMVASTATIN 40MG	50% NEW AS SIMVASTATIN 40MG	100% NEW AS SIMVASTATIN 40MG
2005/06	£78 868	£197 171	£394 341	£788 682
2006/07	£151 236	£378 091	£756 182	£1 512 364
2007/08	£241 695	£604 238	£1 208 475	£2 416 950
Total	£471 800	£1 179 499	£2 358 998	£4 717 996

Underlying data: *PPA*

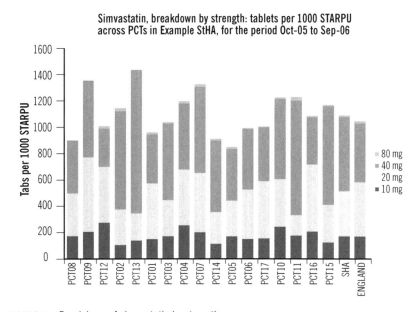

Simvastatin, breakdown by strength: tablets per 1000 STARPU across PCTs in Example StHA, for the period Oct-05 to Sep-06

FIGURE 8.3 Breakdown of simvastatin by strength

However, this is not the whole story. The most evidence-based dose of simvastatin is the 40mg strength. If you look at Figure 8.3 (breakdown of simvastatin by strength), we can see that simvastatin is prescribed at different strengths, so it is possible to work out the extra cost from upgrading all the doses to 40mg tablets (*see* Table 8.2).

TABLE 8.2 Modelled costs of increasing patient dose of simvastatin from 10mg and 20 mg to simvastatin 40mg

| YEAR | EXTRA COST FROM UPGRADING SIMVASTATIN TABLETS TO 40MG STRENGTH | | | |
	10% SWITCH TO SIMVASTATIN 40MG	25% SWITCH TO SIMVASTATIN 40MG	50% SWITCH TO SIMVASTATIN 40MG	100% SWITCH TO SIMVASTATIN 40MG
2005/06	£24 583	£61 457	£122 913	£245 827
2006/07	£29 848	£74 619	£149 238	£298 475
2007/08	£36 843	£92 107	£184 214	£368 428
Total	**£91 273**	**£228 182**	**£456 365**	**£912 730**

Underlying data: *PPA*

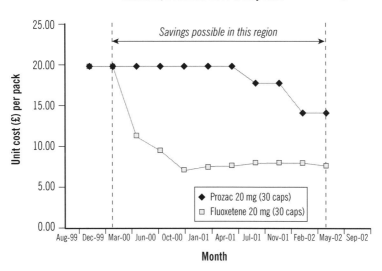

Quarterly price trends (per pack) for branded/unbranded fluoxetine, December 1999 to May 2002

FIGURE 8.4 Price trends (per pack) for Prozac and fluoxetine

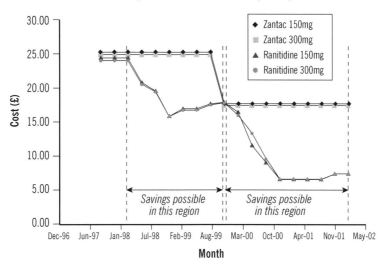

FIGURE 8.5 Trends for branded/unbranded ranitidine costs, September 1997–March 2002 (quarterly)

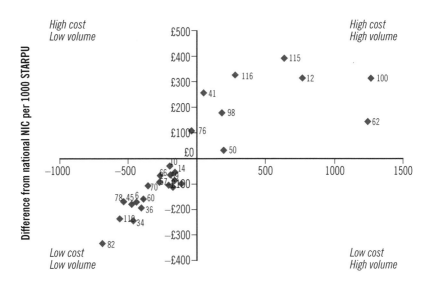

FIGURE 8.6 Boston matrix of antibiotic drug prescribing

The extra costs of implementing the 40mg dose are more than offset by the use of generic simvastatin. Thus a prescriber, or a practice as a whole, can use PACT data to help with cost-minimisation decisions, and balance these against investment costs.

These models are by their nature dynamic. Up until 2005, when medicines came off patent, the drug tariff price (i.e. the price the dispensing pharmacists is dispensed at, i.e. the cost attributed to the prescriber) has reduced at variable rates (Figures 8.4 and 8.5). The new maximum generic pricing scheme should now even out such variations.

The problem with PACT data is also, in a way, its strength.[1] Because the dataset is universal and comprehensive there are vast amounts of data. In a busy day there is little time for the average prescriber to set about the preceding sort of analyses. In some cases practices employ pharmacists or technicians to undertake this work for them, or the information is supplied to them by primary care trusts, who in turn employ pharmacists for this purpose.

Occasionally, as in the West Midlands, an academic unit collects the data on behalf of the PCTs and practices, and turns it into bespoke reports at practice or PCT level. This allows for more sophisticated modelling and the use of other databases to complement and enhance the information that comes from PACT data. For instance, combining the cost and volume data for prescribing of antibiotics onto a Boston matrix (Figure 8.6) allows one to 'quadrant' the practices within a PCT into four categories – high volume, high cost prescribers; high volume, low cost prescribers; low volume, low cost and low volume, high cost.

This also demonstrates the strengths and weaknesses of PACT data referred to in Chapter 7 – it is tempting to assume that the GPs in the top right-hand quadrant who prescribe a lot of antibiotics at high unit costs are 'bad prescribers'. This is a flawed assumption. Without knowing the morbidity of the population they are dealing with, it is impossible to say whether this prescribing is appropriate or not. What it does do, though, is allow for intelligent questioning of the practice via an adviser's visit.

'Mind the gap' – disparities between primary and secondary care

Initially, there was a difference in funding between medicines used in hospitals and those in primary care. Hospital medicines had to be paid for, and budgeted for, in the overall hospital management budget. In primary care, drugs were treated as a separate budget line and for many years enjoyed automatic access to the treasury reserve.

In other words, if hospitals overspent, they had to somehow find a way of recouping their overspend in the next financial year, whereas if the drugs bill was overspent in primary care, the money came from treasury reserves without any immediate sanctions. If adjustments were made for primary care budgets this was spread across the entire national budget, thus the effect of overspending by a particular health authority or cohort of prescribers was diluted nationally and therefore unnoticed by the majority.

A consequence of this was that high unit cost hospital drugs were recommended by specialists, who wrote discharge letters asking GPs to subsequently prescribe the drug. This meant the drug cost shifted from secondary to primary care. With an unwelcome congruence, this also fitted with the pharmaceutical company promotional strategies.

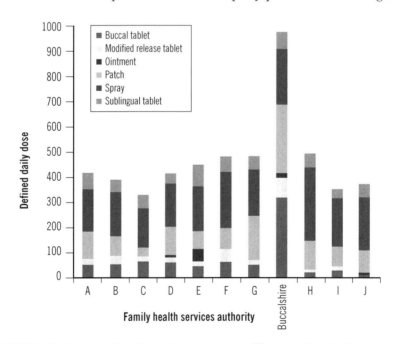

FIGURE 8.7 Relative prescribing of buccal nitrates between different health authorities

Companies relied on key opinion leaders, such as hospital specialists, to choose their drugs and then recommend them to their colleagues in primary care. This could produce quite startling shifts in primary care prescribing. An example of this is the prescribing of buccal nitrate tablets.[2] Figure 8.7 shows the relative prescribing of buccal nitrates between several health authorities. It is tempting to assume this could be down to a difference in incidence of disease, but further analysis showed this not to be the case.

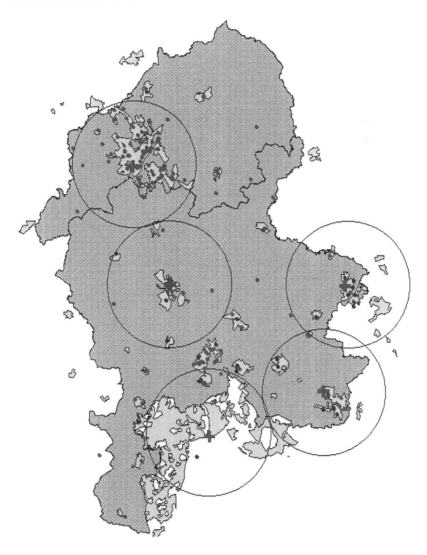

FIGURE 8.8 Prescribing of buccal nitrates in West Midlands Health Authorities

In fact, as Figure 8.8 shows, the high prescribing was clustered in practices surrounding one particular hospital. This turned out to be a consequence of the prescribing of one individual cardiologist. The interesting point is that although this could be monitored in primary care, the cardiologist had no idea of the impact of his own recommendations once patients left hospital.

Hospital data remains a difficult area for economic analyses. It is fine when constructing bespoke economic arguments inside the context of a clinical trial, but there is as yet no universal system for collecting hospital data for health services purposes. At the time of writing, a recent agreement between IMS and the National Health Service may help by bringing more data to light. Area Prescribing Committees, or specialist committees such as the Midlands Therapeutic Review and Advisory Committee (MTRAC), have the remit of managing some of these interface issues.

Combining prescribing and morbidity data

So far, we have only dealt with a simple economic tool, cost-minimisation, and touched on the issues of cost-effectiveness. The example of antibiotic prescribing in Figure 8.6 shows the dangers of making assumptions about prescribing in the absence of data on morbidity. The issue for the health service is that morbidity data has

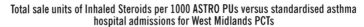

Total sale units of Inhaled Steroids per 1000 ASTRO PUs versus standardised asthma hospital admissions for West Midlands PCTs

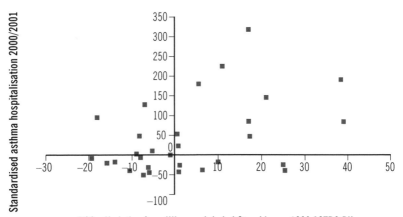

FIGURE 8.9 Inhaled steroids matrix

until recently not been routinely available to the prescriber or the health economy in a format that can be easily accessed and processed. Our experience at Keele has been that by combining datasets, although we can provide no definitive answers, we can move the agenda on by compiling some basic prescribing datasets with proxy measures of morbidity. A recent example is shown in Figure 8.9.

Firstly we used a geographical information system to map out prescribing patterns for corticosteroid reliever inhalers for asthma by post code, then produced a similar map for admissions to hospital for asthma. By comparing the two maps you can take a particular district and look to see if in areas where there is high prescribing this is also high morbidity, or the converse. However, this does involve switching between the two maps and making an intuitive judgement. By combining the data onto a Boston matrix, this time by using morbidity against volume prescribing rather than cost against volume prescribing, we come up with a matrix such as that in Figure 8.9.

From Figure 8.9, you can for instance see that in the top left-hand quadrant there are high admissions for asthma, but very low prescribing of preventative treatment. Again, such analysis must come with a health warning; the two datasets we are using are disparate so this is not directly cause and effect. A little like the antibiotics graph in Figure 8.6, it does move the discussion further on and if a health economy is deciding where to place scarce advisory or supportive resources, such a matrix is a good start in helping them with that decision-making process.

The recent introduction of the new general practitioner contract with its quality and outcomes framework (QOF), has produced a drug-diagnosis dataset linked at patient level which helps towards being able to understand drug usage more clearly. Under this new contract, GP prescribers are not only paid on a capitation bases, that is on the basis of the number of patients who are registered with them, but are also paid on a points system for intervening with certain groups of patients, and recording both the diagnosis and the outcome. Thus the average GP in the UK should routinely be able to access data on the number of patients that have had a heart attack, and the number of those patients that are being treated with a statin, or vice versa. PCTs should also be able to get these data at aggregated level.

It is early days yet, but it should be possible to transmute the data from the Quality Management and Analysis System (QMAS) onto the sort of Boston matrices that have previously been used using proxy measures of morbidity. Whilst a welcome significant change, there are still some disadvantages to this dataset, in particular the issue of timing – because the GP can enter the data any time during the financial year, then the dataset will only be valid at the end of that financial year. Thus although it is effective for remunerating GPs for meeting their QOF targets, from an epidemiological point of view it will be some time before we are able to build a robust dataset from annual data points. From an economic point of view it may help with financial forecasts based on disease prevalence estimates from QOF, e.g. estimating the number of patients with coronary heart disease not currently being treated to target.

Data to support national economic appraisal

It is not only individual prescribers who are blighted by an inability to link prescribing and morbidity data at the individual patient level. Both the major sets of guidance in England and Wales, the National Institute for Health and Clinical Excellence (NICE) and the National Service Frameworks (NSFs) provide clear and specific guidance on the use of medicines. Unfortunately, for the health service, this national guidance is often conditional; it recommends the use of a drug in some circumstances but not in others. For instance the NSF for coronary heart disease has a target for lipid lowering drugs being used in secondary prevention, that is, after a heart attack. It is impossible from PACT data alone to discern whether the increased use in statins is for this purpose or whether it is being used for primary prevention. QMAS data from the QOF should help here. Unfortunately, the GP contract only covers very specific areas, and NICE guidance covers a variety of therapeutic groups. Currently, at the best, all we can do routinely is show increases or decreases in prescribing. If NICE says no to a product, from a governance point of view this is simple – there should be no more prescriptions, which can be simply monitored by using PACT data. If the verdict is conditional – say for a particular diagnosis, then routine data cannot discern if any increase is appropriate. Furthermore, any change may be masked inside the overall trends; for instance, prior to the withdrawal from the market of COX-II (a selective anti-inflammatory non-steroidal drug) inhibitors, it was difficult to discern any change resulting from NICE guidance, as overall prescribing was increasing at a steady rate. This means surveys and samples and more sophisticated modelling as used by Sheldon *et al.* are necessary,[3] which although they demonstrate a change, are far too labour-intensive for routine monitoring.

What next?

Recent reorganisations within the NHS, in particular the advent of practice-based commissioning groups, have brought investment and disinvestment decisions back to the level of large practices or groups of practices. Whilst this is remarkably like fundholding, there are now some fundamental differences. We have national guidance on key disease areas, benchmarks for practices to be audited against, and a national body to audit these standards. In addition we have a national body, NICE, to determine the value for money of interventions with medicines and devices. The central health economic decisions are now made using complex modelling driven by traditional clinical trial data and some limited naturalistic studies.

At a local level the easy savings are no longer there – generic prescribing rates in the UK are on average over 70%, in contrast to rates as low as 30% in the early days of fundholding. Value for money will therefore be more a case of careful selection of agents within a class, or one class of agents instead of another, for treating a condition. The recent ASCOT trial[4] perhaps exemplifies this; the results are used by marketers as recommending calcium channel blockers and ACE inhibitors over thiazide diuretics, whereas careful appraisal suggests this may not be the case. Understanding current usage using PACT will be essential to estimate the economic impact of changing practice policy to act on studies such as ASCOT. In addition the QMAS data will help give a perspective on relative burden of disease, and will prioritise activity in these areas. Whilst quality data remains the cornerstone of practices forming such policies, intelligent and critical interpretation of both the data and the context in which it is applied will be essential, which can only be done with the full co-operation of multidisciplinary teams. Individualised care, and the emphasis on proper diagnosis and care of the patient, and their understanding of that care, is quite properly at the heart of policy, but increasingly practices may now start to use the data at their disposal to engage in a more reflective consideration of the resources at their disposal, and engage in more of a public health approach to the management of their patient population.

Conclusion

Routine datasets can be, and have been, used for making decisions at PCO level using basic health economic principles. However, the limitations of these decisions, due to the inherent constraints within the data, are widely acknowledged. Future developments must include intelligent and critical understanding of how to interpret the data, and exploration of linkage across different datasets such as prescribing and morbidity. As medical records become more interactive and comprehensive, decisions will increasingly be informed on the basis of individualised care which will be auditable through analysis of routine data.

References

1. Chapman S. Prescribing information systems: making sense of primary care data. *J Clinical Pharmacy and Therapeutics* 2001; **26**: 235–9.
2. Pryce A, Chapman SR, Heatlie H. Buccaling under the pressure: do secondary care establishments influence primary care prescribing? *BMJ* 1996; **313**: 1621–4.
3. Sheldon TA, Cullum N, Dawson D, Lanksheer A, Lowson K, Watt I *et al.* What's the evidence that NICE guidance has been implemented? Results from a national evaluation using time series analysis, audit of patients' notes, and interviews. *BMJ* 2004; **329**: 999–1004.
4. ASCOT (Anglo-Scandinavian Cardiac Outcomes Trial) http://ascotstudy.org/ (accessed 26 August 2007).

9 Pharmacovigilance

DEBORAH LAYTON AND ANTHONY COX

This chapter discusses the background to the need for pharma-covigilance and describes in detail two of the main mechanisms by which this is studied in the UK: the Yellow Card Spontaneous Reporting Scheme, and Prescription-Event Monitoring. A brief discussion of the complementarity of the two systems concludes this chapter.

Introduction

In order to market a drug, pharmaceutical companies have to demonstrate efficacy and provide evidence of safety of their product. However, it is not possible to discover the complete safety profile of a new drug prior to its launch. Clinical trials of a new drug test the drug on an average of around 2500 patients in total, with fewer than a hundred patients using the drug for longer than a year.[1,2] Patients within trials are often relatively healthy, without the multiple disease states or complex drug histories of real world patients. Rare and potentially serious adverse effects can remain undetected until the drug is used in a larger population.

Although predictable adverse events may be identified in clinical trials, the first suspicions of a less common or unpredictable reaction may often be seen in a case report from a practitioner. However, the time it takes a vigilant doctor to publish a suspected adverse reaction in the literature, even if accepted for publication, could be many months, during which further patients may be exposed to the potential risk.

Pharmacovigilance is concerned with detection, assessment and prevention of adverse effects or any other possible drug related problems, with the ultimate goal of achieving rational and safe therapeutic decisions in clinical practice. There are many sources of data for the process of pharmacovigilance in the United Kingdom (UK), and this chapter describes two co-existing and complementary pharmacovigilance systems. These are a spontaneous reporting system used in the UK called the Yellow Card Scheme, and a targeted system known as Prescription-Event Monitoring.

The Commission on Human Medicines (CHM), an advisory committee to the Medicines and Healthcare Products Regulatory Authority (MHRA), requests notifications of all *suspected* adverse drug reactions (ADR) from newly approved products and *serious* ADRs for established drugs and vaccines, through the 'Yellow Card' reporting scheme. Prescription-Event Monitoring (PEM) is the only national scheme available to all general practitioners, in addition to the Yellow Card Scheme, and aims to monitor the safety of recently marketed medicines, under the conditions of general practice in England.

The Yellow Card Spontaneous Reporting Scheme at the Medicines and Healthcare Products Regulatory Agency

Background

As has been noted in other chapters, severe ADRs associated with the drug thalidomide were a turning point for drug safety within the UK. Introduced originally in West Germany in 1956, thalidomide was marketed in 1958 in the United Kingdom as Distaval®. A successful marketing campaign led to wide prescribing of the drug. First suspicions of a serious problem were raised in November 1961, after investigations at obstetric units in West Germany showed a large rise in the number of children born with limb deformities. By the time thalidomide was withdrawn, over 10,000 babies had been born deformed.

As a result of this appalling human toll, attention focused on the adverse reactions of all drugs. Many countries established drug regulatory bodies to ensure adequate testing of drugs before marketing and pharmacovigilance systems to monitor their safety after marketing. In the UK this took the form of the formation of the advisory body the Committee on Safety of Drugs. One of the responsibilities of this committee was to collect and disseminate information relating to adverse effects of drugs. In May 1964 the Yellow Card Scheme was launched within the United Kingdom.

The Committee on Safety of Drugs later became The Committee on Safety of Medicines (CSM). On 30 November 2005, the CSM was replaced by The Commission on Human Medicines (CHM). The scheme continues to be administered by the CHM and MHRA.

The Yellow Card Scheme

The Yellow Card Scheme was established with four key principles,[3]

1 Suspected adverse reactions should be reported; reporters do not need to be certain or prove that the drug caused the reaction.
2 It is the responsibility of all doctors and dentists to report.
3 Reporters should report without delay.
4 Reports could be made and would be treated in confidence.

In 1969 coroners were admitted to the scheme. Attempts to increase the size of the reporter base in the recent years have led to the extension of the scheme to hospital pharmacists,[4] community pharmacists[5] and nurses.[6]

Reports to the Yellow Card Scheme are made on yellow reporting forms available in the *British National Formulary*, *The British Dental Formulary*, MIMS, from regional Yellow Card centres and direct from the MHRA via a freephone number. Reports can also be submitted electronically at http://www.yellowcard.gov.uk.

Over the years the reporting card has been redesigned as the level of information required has changed. In 2000, a revision of the General Medical Council's guidelines on confidentiality led to the anonymisation of the Yellow Card Scheme. Reporters are advised now only to provide a local identification number, initials and the patient's age, rather than a patient's name, date of birth or NHS number.

In April of 2004 an Independent Review of the Yellow Card Scheme was published.[7] The report was published on the fortieth anniversary of the scheme, and was highly supportive of the original principles of the Yellow Card Scheme. It also heralded important changes in the dissemination of collected data proposing a significant opening up of access to the database.

What should be reported?

Any suspected reaction to the following groups of agents should be reported, no matter how trivial:

1. Drugs and vaccines that are being closely monitored (indicated by a black triangle '▼' in the British National Formulary).
2. Any drug used in a child.
3. Any herbal preparation.

For established products, any suspected serious reactions should be reported. Serious reactions include those that are fatal, life-threatening, disabling, incapacitating or which result in or prolong hospitalisation and/or are medically significant. Congenital abnormalities following drug use are also classified as serious. A copy of a yellow card is given in Figure 9.1.

The methodology

Statistical methods for detecting signals of ADRs in a database of spontaneously collected reports will be described later in this chapter, but it is important to note that the Yellow Card Scheme is only one of many methods used by the MHRA to identify safety issues.

Over half a million Yellow Card reports collected since 1964 were stored in a database known as the Adverse Drug Reaction On-line Information Tracking (ADROIT) system. In May of 2006, the database was transferred to a new MHRA information management system called Sentinel.

Reports are coded onto the database by scientific staff and undergo a number of quality assurance steps to maintain a high standard of data. Scanned images of the original reports are stored on the system.

The combination of patient-anonymous reports and an increase in the size of the reporter base means that duplicate reports are possible, and potentially more difficult to discover. The Sentinel system is able to identify duplicate reports and pools the information from multiple reports of the same reaction.

A crucial part of any reporting scheme is the classification of adverse reactions within the database. The MHRA use the *Medical Dictionary for Regulatory Activities* (MedDRA), a structured dictionary of medical terms adopted as an international standard by the International Conference on Harmonisation.[8]

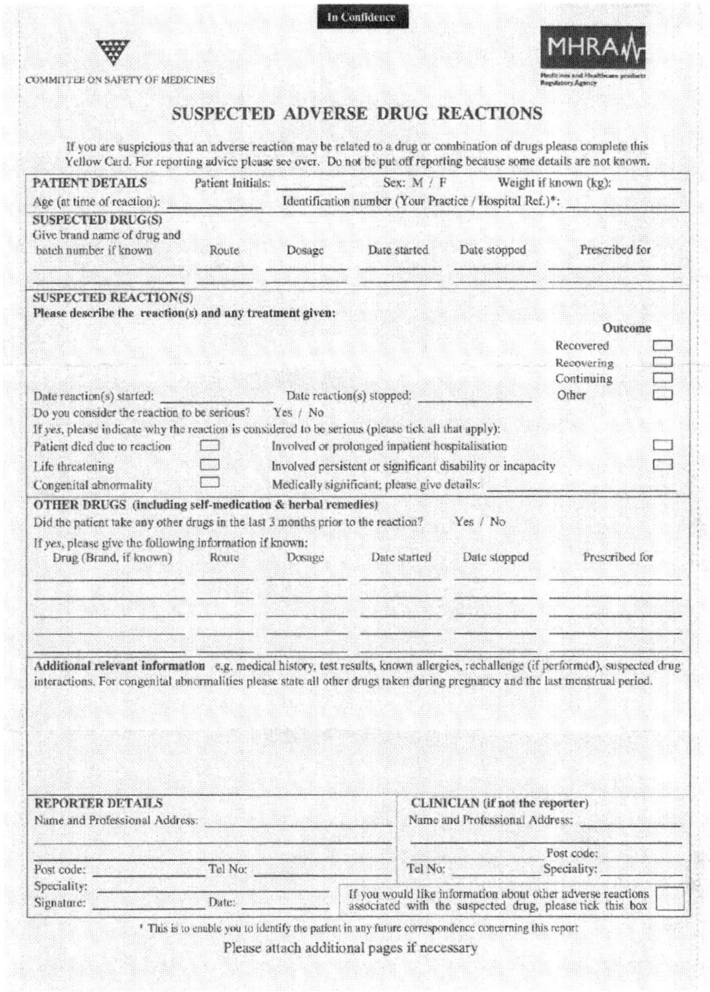

In Confidence

COMMITTEE ON SAFETY OF MEDICINES

MHRA

Medicines and Healthcare products Regulatory Agency

SUSPECTED ADVERSE DRUG REACTIONS

If you are suspicious that an adverse reaction may be related to a drug or combination of drugs please complete this Yellow Card. For reporting advice please see over. Do not be put off reporting because some details are not known.

PATIENT DETAILS   Patient Initials: _____   Sex: M / F   Weight if known (kg): _____
Age (at time of reaction): _____   Identification number (Your Practice / Hospital Ref.)*: _____

SUSPECTED DRUG(S)
Give brand name of drug and
batch number if known   Route   Dosage   Date started   Date stopped   Prescribed for

SUSPECTED REACTION(S)
Please describe the reaction(s) and any treatment given:

Outcome
Recovered ☐
Recovering ☐
Continuing ☐
Other ☐

Date reaction(s) started: _____   Date reaction(s) stopped: _____
Do you consider the reaction to be serious?   Yes / No
If yes, please indicate why the reaction is considered to be serious (please tick all that apply):
Patient died due to reaction ☐   Involved or prolonged inpatient hospitalisation ☐
Life threatening ☐   Involved persistent or significant disability or incapacity ☐
Congenital abnormality ☐   Medically significant; please give details: _____

OTHER DRUGS (including self-medication & herbal remedies)
Did the patient take any other drugs in the last 3 months prior to the reaction?   Yes / No

If yes, please give the following information if known:
Drug (Brand, if known)   Route   Dosage   Date started   Date stopped   Prescribed for

Additional relevant information e.g. medical history, test results, known allergies, rechallenge (if performed), suspected drug interactions. For congenital abnormalities please state all other drugs taken during pregnancy and the last menstrual period.

REPORTER DETAILS
Name and Professional Address: _____

Post code: _____   Tel No: _____
Speciality: _____
Signature: _____   Date: _____

CLINICIAN (if not the reporter)
Name and Professional Address: _____
Post code: _____
Tel No: _____   Speciality: _____

If you would like information about other adverse reactions associated with the suspected drug, please tick this box ☐

* This is to enable you to identify the patient in any future correspondence concerning this report

Please attach additional pages if necessary

FIGURE 9.1 The Yellow Card

Strengths and weaknesses of the Yellow Card Scheme

Spontaneous ADR reporting systems such as the Yellow Card Scheme are regarded as the classic drug safety alert ('signalling') system and their major purpose is to provide early warnings of possible hazards from use of medicines. Such systems are relatively cheap to operate and provide continuous safety monitoring throughout the lifespan of a medicinal product. In the Yellow Card Scheme, over 70% of reports come directly from UK healthcare professionals. The system is confidential and reporters may submit reports without fear of litigation. In other systems, such as the American MedWatch Scheme, the majority of reports are received through pharmaceutical companies. The scheme also examines the use of drugs in a large and varied population with regard to sex, disease states and concomitant medication, which enables the MHRA to obtain information about factors which may predispose to ADRs.

Spontaneous reporting schemes have a number of limitations. Schemes suffer from under-reporting, which is variable in nature.[9] Around 6% of all potentially reportable reactions may be reported to the Yellow Card Scheme.[10] The reporting rates for suspected reactions of a serious nature, or to a new drug under intense surveillance, may be higher.[11] In recent years increasing pressures on GPs appear to have affected the level of GP reporting.[12] Spontaneous reporting schemes are passive surveillance systems; reliance is placed on the ability of health professionals to recognise possible ADRs and to distinguish these from symptoms related to the underlying disease. With regard to quantifying the risk, such systems supply a numerator (the number of reports) but estimates of the incidence of reactions cannot be made, because the measure of the population exposed cannot be ascertained accurately. These factors and other strengths and limitations are discussed in detail elsewhere.[13]

A number of initiatives have been undertaken to maintain the Yellow Card Scheme profile and to promote reporting. Some of these are listed below:

Extension of the Yellow Card Scheme to other professionals

As noted already, hospital pharmacists, community pharmacists, nurses, midwives and health visitors are now valid reporters to the Yellow Card Scheme, and efforts to develop the reporting culture within these professions have been encouraged in addition to the original professions allowed to report.

Internet reporting

The lack of availability of Yellow Cards has been cited as a reason for not reporting. As computers become more widely used in the healthcare environment, electronic reporting may become a useful method of capturing formerly unreported reactions. The MHRA has established the website http://www.yellowcard.gov.uk which provides an online ADR submission form and guidance on reporting.

The HIV ADR reporting scheme

The HIV ADR reporting scheme is an extension of the Yellow Card Scheme. Reports are made on blue cards. Its aim is to promote knowledge about the safety of drugs used in HIV patients and to encourage reporting. The scheme is a collaboration between the MHRA and the Medicines Research Council Clinical Trials Unit.

Herbal Safety News

In 2003, the MHRA launched a new information service on its website dedicated to providing up to date safety information on herbal medicines for the public, herbalists, the herbal industry and health professionals. It is hoped that the service will increase understanding that herbal remedies are genuine medicines, should be manufactured to the same high standards as conventional medicines and subjected to the same monitoring processes. The site will include issues such as: details of herbal remedies found to be interacting with other medicines (e.g. St John's wort and its interaction with prescription medicines), inherent safety concerns of an ingredient itself (e.g. kava-kava may on rare occasions be associated with liver toxicity), confusion over potent herbal ingredients and contamination or adulteration of herbal remedies with heavy metals or prescription only medicines. *Herbal Safety News* is available at the MHRA website (http://www.mhra.gov.uk).

Should ADR reporting be made a legal requirement or attract a fee?

Reporting to the UK Yellow Card Scheme is a voluntary activity. In some countries, such as Sweden, the reporting of ADRs to their equivalent scheme is a legal requirement. However, reporting rates to the UK's Yellow Card Scheme are higher than those in countries with a legal obligation. Medical confidentiality also means that enforcement of such a law is practically impossible; there is currently no government interest in changing the voluntary nature of the scheme. The Independent Review of the Yellow Card Scheme did not endorse payments for reporting, although some have argued that payments linked to targets for reporting could increase reporting.

Dissemination of drug safety information from the Yellow Card Scheme

Feedback to companies

The MHRA is under a legal obligation to provide information to manufacturers of medicinal products. Increasingly the MHRA is focused on developing more efficient information systems for rapid electronic transfer of information. In the past, the ADROIT Electronically Generated Information System (AEGIS), introduced in 1993, enabled the rapid electronic exchange of information between the pharmaceutical industry and the MHRA. Following the decommissioning of the ADROIT and the AEGIS system, and the move to the Sentinel system, some companies have had problems developing electronic links to the MHRA. As an interim solution those companies download data via a portal at the MHRA website, until the ultimate aim of all companies receiving data electronically has been achieved.

Companies are provided with restricted access to anonymous data about their products on the database. The type of information provided includes the following:

- Drug Analysis Prints (DAPs) – These consist of a summary of all suspected ADRs reported to have occurred in association with a named drug substance marketed within the UK.
- Product Analysis Prints (PAPs) – A summary print of all suspected ADRs reported to have occurred in association with a named product.
- Anonymised Single Patient Prints (ASPPs) – Anonymous case of an ADR report.
- Reaction Analysis Prints (RAPs) – A listing of all drug substances associated with a particular adverse reaction term.
- Fatal reports – A cumulative analysis of the cause of death reported on ADR reports for a specific substance.

The MHRA also provides an ad hoc query service for the industry.

Feedback to reporters

All reporters to the Yellow Card Scheme receive an acknowledgement of their report. When filling in their Yellow Card reporters have the option of ticking a box for further information. If ticked they will be sent a DAP of reactions within the Sentinel database to the suspected drug. A DAP lists all reactions reported to have occurred in association with the named suspect drug. Since a Yellow Card report may contain more than one reaction, the DAP will contain more reactions than Yellow Card reports. Data are included for the multi-constituent products as well as single products. ADRs are listed in a hierarchical structure (Figure 9.2). The date of the earliest reaction is listed, as well as the date that the data was extracted.

There are some important guidance points, made available by the MHRA, about the interpretation of the DAPs as follows.

- Reports are suspected reactions, not proven reactions. The listing of a reaction with a drug does not in itself provide evidence of causality.
- Medicines are commonly used in combination. For example many vaccines are used in combination. It can be difficult to ascribe a suspected reaction to an individual vaccine or drug.
- Certain conditions can occur spontaneously without a drug being administered. If a drug is used in a large population there may be co-incidental temporal relationships leading to an ADR report.
- The reactions do not give a basis for determining the incidence of any reaction. The exact number of reactions is unknown due to

SYSTEM ORGAN CLASS HIGH LEVEL TERM	SINGLE CONST		MULTI CONST	
REACTION NAME	TOT	FTL	TOT	FTL
Hepatocellular damage				
Hepatocellular damage NOS	1	0	0	0
Hepatorenal syndrome	1	1	0	0
Liver fatty	4	0	0	0
Jaundice (all forms)				
Jaundice NOS	13	0	0	0
Jaundice cholestatic	4	1	0	0
Jaundice hepatocellular	1	0	0	0
Sys Organ Class Total	102	2	0	0

SINGLE CONST = Reactions involving a single constituent product; MULTI CONST = Reactions involving a multi-constituent product; TOT = number of reactions; FTL = number of those reactions that were fatal; NOS = Not otherwise specified.

FIGURE 9.2 Extract of Drug Analysis Print from MHRA

under-reporting, and the total number of patients using the drug is not known.

■ Numerical comparisons cannot be made between different drugs, on the basis of a DAP report. Comparisons are misleading since they do not take account of the variations in ADR reporting, the extent of the use of a drug and other confounding variables such as the channelling of high-risk patients towards drugs perceived as safer than others.

Printed materials

Safety bulletins can be an extremely useful tool, if well distributed. In the past doctors, dentists, coroners and pharmacists received *Current Problems in Pharmacovigilance* published by the now defunct CSM. This bulletin published the outcomes of regulatory decisions, advice to prescribers and new safety concerns. Some of these safety messages are also found in the relevant sections of the *British National Formulary*. The increase in the reporter base (in particular the admission of a large number of nurse reporters) led to discussion about additional and more effective methods of dissemination of safety messages. *Current Problems in Pharmacovigilance* used to be published three to four times a year, but from 2004 to 2006 only two editions were published. In August 2007 the MHRA replaced Current Problems in *Pharmacovigilance* with a monthly electronic publication entitled *Drug Safety Update*. The journal is intended for all UK healthcare professionals.

Other publications by the MHRA include 'Dear Doctor/health professional letters' which are cascaded throughout the healthcare system to highlight important safety issues that require urgent attention.

The MHRA website

The MHRA website at www.mhra.gov.uk is an increasingly important aid in distributing drug safety information. As well as publishing electronic versions of *Current Problems in Pharmacovigilance*, and general information about the MHRA and CHM, the MHRA website has a rolling front page that carries recent news and link to other relevant sites. The use of the website to provide much wider access to the reports, resulting from the 2004 review of the scheme, is discussed in more detail below.

The Independent Review of Access to the Yellow Card Scheme

The primary purpose of the review was to identify the conditions under which whole datasets from the individual Yellow Card Scheme might be released, given the increased pressure from external researchers and the pharmaceutical industry for greater access to the Yellow Card database. Although it was expected that most requests would be for subsets of the data, others might wish to have access to the entire database for signal detection methods. A major concern was that such data could be misinterpreted if the limitations of the data were not recognised, and false conclusions might be reached about safety and adverse effects on public health. However, given that the prime purpose of the Yellow Card database is the detection of important drug safety signals, it was considered unethical not to allow greater access. Refusal could also be seen as being obstructive and against the interests of drug safety.

As well as the dangers of misinterpretation and misunderstanding from independent analyses, concern was expressed by some groups during the consultation period that the Yellow Card data might be used for purposes not expressed when the scheme was founded. However, there was wide support for optimising the use of the Yellow Card data for research and public health, so long as it did not deter reporting. It was also considered essential that patients should have the confidence that their identity and personal data would not be disclosed for research purposes without consent.

The review divided the data into three categories:

Set I: Aggregated anonymous-identifiable data excluding all patient and reporter details.

Set II: Information held within individual Yellow Cards, excluding patient and reporter identifiable data.

Set III: Information from the Yellow Card, with an opportunity for obtaining further information from the reporter.

It was recommended that Category I data should be published regularly on the MHRA website. The frequency of publication was not specified, but the committee suggested that the rate at which the data profile changes and the observation that frequent feedback improves reporting of ADRs should be borne in mind. The committee felt that publishing all aggregated and unidentifiable Yellow Card Scheme data for all drugs in the UK would be an 'enormous task'. Currently, the MHRA have a selection of DAPs available on their website for download, along with advice on interpretation of the material. Aggregated anonymous-identifiable data not provided on the website is available on request under the Freedom of Information Act.

The MHRA will not release data where there are five or fewer reports about a particular ADR, due to concerns about patient and reporter confidentiality. For the same reasons, the number of reports submitted to the Yellow Card Scheme by individual hospitals or primary care trusts will not be released.

The committee advised that research proposals that involve access to individual Yellow Card reports in categories II and III should be subject to independent scientific and ethical scrutiny by appropriate bodies. Some category II data proposals could avoid scientific and ethical review if they fulfilled a set of criteria established by the scientific committee.

Even though category III data allows contact with the reporter, the anonymity of both the reporter and the patients remains important, with further details not being obtained without consent from the patient, and the MHRA as an initial contact with the reporter, in order to ask for consent to pass on their details to any researcher.

All requests not covered by FOI will be assessed by an independent scientific committee set up by the MHRA. All proposals will have the same set of rules regardless of origin. Straightforward applications that satisfy previously agreed criteria may avoid the full scrutiny of the independent scientific committee. No patient details or patient identifiers should be released. Requests outside of the Freedom of Information Act will have a scale of charges for access to the data.

Yellow Card centres

While the Yellow Card scheme is centrally administered by the MHRA at a national level, five regional Yellow Card centres (YCCs) exist in the United Kingdom: West Midlands, Mersey, Northern and Yorkshire, Wales, and Scotland. YCCs were established in order to stimulate ADR reporting, to improve communication, answer queries and provide information about ADR reporting to reporters at a local level, often through the publication of local drug safety bulletins. YCCs are usually based within local medicines information centres or university departments of clinical pharmacology; the local contact and expert advice provided to clinical colleagues in regions by clinical pharmacologists and pharmacists employed by YCCs is particularly valued. Additional roles undertaken by YCCs include the provision of educational events about ADR reporting and the Yellow Card Scheme, as well as undertaking research within the area of ADRs and drug safety. All YCCs have websites reachable from the main MHRA website or http://www.yellowcard.gov.uk.

The Independent Review of Access to the Yellow Card Scheme advised that YCCs needed to be more closely integrated with the Yellow Card Scheme. In the past, Yellow Cards sent to YCCs were transcribed into local databases and forwarded to the MHRA. The report argued that all Yellow Cards should be collated centrally, with copies of Yellow Cards being returned to the relevant YCC. Concerns were expressed that this may disconnect the YCCs from their reporting base, and lose the local element of the scheme. However, from April 2006, all Yellow Cards were collected centrally, with YCCs being supplied with information to follow up local reports if further information is required from a reporter. Given the review's support for the educational role of YCCs, it is expected their information provision and educational roles will expand. Existing YCCs may extend their coverage to other areas, and additional YCCs may be formed.

External views of the Yellow Card Scheme

The Yellow Card Scheme has in recent years come under scrutiny from the National Audit Office (NAO),[14] the Public Accounts Committee of Parliament,[15] and more recently the Independent Review on Access to the Yellow Card Scheme.[7] Although all have recognised the valuable contribution the MHRA has made to public health, some points were made about the operation of the Yellow Card Scheme.

The NAO suggested that the MHRA should build on its existing regional networks and work with others such as hospital and community pharmacists and consultants, in order to aid the dissemi-nation of key information on medicines safety to health professionals. The public accounts committee noted that efforts to improve reporting rates were seen to have met limited success. The committee also found that the MHRA had a narrow view of its public role and no public profile. Even among doctors, there was limited awareness of its role. The MHRA was asked to look at the possibilities of patient reporting; The Independent Review on Access to the Yellow Card Scheme also supported this view, advising that patients should be allowed to directly report to the Yellow Card Scheme.

Patient reporting of ADRs

Increasing patient awareness, and changes in the professional patient relationship, combined with pressure from consumer groups means that the argument for patient reporting cannot be ignored. The gateway role that professionals hold at present gives an impression of 'filtering' reactions that the public considers important. This leaves regulatory authorities open to the accusation that they do not consider public concerns.

Existing pharmacovigilance systems and methods focus on health professional reporters' suspicions, which whilst unproven are grounded in clinical experience. By patients submitting directly to the regulatory authority, their reports will not be 'filtered' through the healthcare professional (who may themselves introduce bias based on their own expectations and interpretations of what is credible, serious, and relevant and worth reporting). Thus, whilst patient reporting might provide useful data on their personal experiences, it could also lead to difficulty in separating important signals from background noise, i.e. too much data, with the associated danger that patient reporting may become a drain on an overstretched pharmacovigilance system. Given the known under-reporting of suspected ADRs by health professionals,[9] the aforementioned filtering process between the patient and the regulatory bodies might well be preventing important reactions being reported. Therefore the logical outcome of this situation is that patient reports should be accepted to help combat this situation. Patients may also report reactions to off-label use of drugs, and/or the use of herbal or over the counter medicines – an area that regulatory bodies currently obtain little information about.

Supporters suggest that patient reporting may discover safety signals earlier than healthcare professional reporting. A small study in the Netherlands found patients reported ADRs seven months earlier than professionals,[16] but at present the evidence is equivocal.[17] Patient reports may also be more susceptible to media scare stories resulting in a bias in patient reporting.

The mechanisms of reporting vary between countries, with some systems requiring validation of a report by a health professional. Initially, the MHRA did not accept direct patient reporting of ADRs. Instead, small pilots of patient reporting were launched with NHS Direct, a telephone health advice system run in the UK in April 2003. In these pilots, patient reports were facilitated through the trained

NHS Direct staff who acted as learned intermediaries. The results were largely disappointing with a limited number of reports, and critical comments from patient groups that the scheme merely transferred the decision to report a reaction from a doctor to a nurse, rather than collecting patients' qualitative experiences. In 2004 The Independent Review of Access to the Yellow Card Scheme recommended that a direct patient reporting system should be introduced. The Chairman of the Steering Committee suggested that patients would not use the conventional scientific or medical language in their reports, but noted that 'on the whole the people who know something is having an adverse effect on their body are the patients'.[18]

Patient reports are likely to differ from professional reports, and this has implications for pharmacovigilance. E-mails elicited in the wake of a BBC current affairs programme (*Panorama*) examining the safety of selective serotonin reuptake inhibitors (SSRIs) were systematically examined for patient experiences.[19] Although most e-mails were deficient in key data, such as name, sex and age of the informant, dosage or duration of treatment, concurrent medication and diagnosis, the collective weight of the reports was judged to be profound, and were felt to provide qualitatively rich experiences of adverse reactions.

The patient reporting scheme of the MHRA was re-launched as a pilot scheme in January 2005, and rolled out nationally in October 2005. It includes an electronic form for reporting ADRs directly rolled out nationally, a telephone number and a paper form which has been made available in a limited number of pilot sites. The form includes fields which attempt to capture basic demographic and drug information, but also allows free typing of the reaction experienced by the patient. In the first year the MHRA received approximately 700 reports, which they considered to be generally of a high quality.[20]

The MHRA's patient reporting scheme will be evaluated in 2007 over a two year period. The evaluation is to look at the patient experience: awareness of the scheme, the effectiveness of communication strategies to encourage reporting, patients' reaction to the scheme and ability to fill in Yellow Cards unaided, and views on the user friendliness, effectiveness and usability of the differing reporting mechanisms. The impact on pharmacovigilance will also be evaluated: the richness of patient descriptions, the time-lag between ADR occurrence and reporting and the relative contribution of patient reporting to signal generation in terms of quantity and quality.[20]

Since under-reporting of ADRs by heath professionals is cited as a concern by the public in drug safety controversies,[21] it is important not to underestimate the potential role patient reporting has in increasing public trust in the safety of drugs, and regulatory bodies such as the MHRA. A patient reporting system also raises an expectation of 'results'; how feedback will be provided remains unclear. Patient reporting is likely to become much more important in the next 10 to 20 years.

Prescription-Event Monitoring at the Drug Safety Research Unit, Southampton

Background

The postmarketing Drug Surveillance Research Unit was set up by Professor William Inman, with financial assistance from the Office of the Chief Scientist of the DHSS, in 1980. Initially part of the Department of Medicine of the University of Southampton, the Unit was reconstituted as a charitable trust in 1986 and its title was altered to the Drug Safety Research Unit (DSRU). The Drug Safety Research Trust is a registered independent charity (No. 327206) operating in association with the University of Portsmouth. Prescription-Event Monitoring (PEM) is conducted in accordance with the International Ethical Guidelines for Biomedical Research prepared by the Council for International Organisations of Medical Science in collaboration with the World Health Organization relating to records based research.[22] It also complies with the Guidelines on the practice of Ethical Committees in Medical Research involving Human Subjects, for records based research, as issued by the Royal College of Physicians.[23] In addition, PEM is listed in the General Medical Council booklet (supplement), *Confidentiality: Protecting and Providing Information*, as 'a professional organisation that monitors the safety of medicines to which doctors should provide relevant information from patients' records wherever possible'.[24] PEM is also included in the report detailing methods in which healthcare professionals can help improve reporting of adverse drug reactions.[12]

Decisions regarding which drugs are to be monitored are reached independently by the DSRU. In general, doctors are not paid to participate, but on a few occasions extraordinary costs of special follow-up enquiries are met from Unit funds. The DSRU looks to the marketing authorisation holders to donate funds in order to cover the costs of the studies undertaken but this is not always achieved.

The methodology

The technique of PEM has been described in detail elsewhere.[25] When a new drug is licensed and selected by the DSRU, the NHS Business Services Authority (NHSBSA) in England is notified (Figure 9.3). Exposure data for the study drug is obtained from data collected on dispensed NHS prescriptions issued by GPs immediately after the date of marketing until a sufficiently large cohort of eligible patients (>30 000) has been identified. The NHSBSA makes available a limited set of data under an agreed protocol to the DSRU. The protocol complies with the requirements of the Data Protection Act (registration No. B0077065). The NHSBSA data is sent to the DSRU in

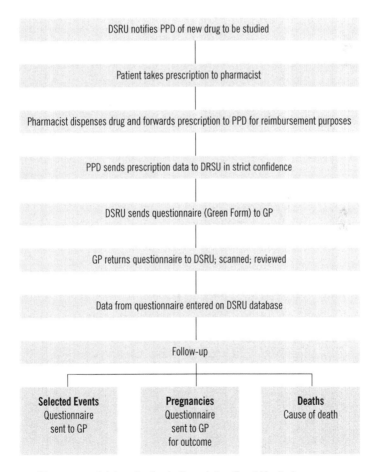

FIGURE 9.3 The process of data collection in Prescription-Event Monitoring (PPD = Prescription Pricing Division of NHS BSA)

confidence to be downloaded onto the PEM database. Demographic and outcome data (event reports) for each patient are obtained by sending simple questionnaires (Green Forms) to the prescribing GP at least six months after the date of the first prescription for each eligible individual patient, until a cohort size of at least 10 000 patients (for whom a Green Form is returned) is achieved. This interim period before the Green Form is sent allows for the newly licensed drug to penetrate the market; prescribing patterns to establish; and collection of NHS prescription data, longitudinal follow-up and sufficient time to achieve anticipated cohort sizes. PEM studies aim to recruit at least 10 000 patients, since this allows one to be 95% certain that any events not observed occur less often than 1 in 3333 cases.[26]

The Green Form questionnaires request information on patient age, indication for prescribing, dose, effectiveness, duration of treatment (start and stop dates), reasons for stopping and any significant health related events the patient experienced since starting the drug. Events are considered to be an ADR if the GP specifies that the event was attributable to the drug. Events attributed to other medication are examined in order to detect possible interactions between the study drug and other concomitant drugs. Reported events are coded using the DSRU event dictionary, a hierarchical dictionary arranged by system-organ class with selective 'lower' terms grouped together under broader 'higher' terms. Green Forms returned with no useful information are classified as 'void' and are excluded from the study and subsequent analysis, as there is no means of determining whether forms not completed indicated no reported events. For some PEM studies, such as the COX-2 inhibitors, rofecoxib and celecoxib, additional questions are included on the Green Form requesting information on potential risk factors in order to address the issue of 'channelling', or preferential prescribing (Figure 9.4).

Each Green Form returned is reviewed by a DSRU research fellow and the context of each event assessed. All pregnancies, any events of medical interest not mentioned in the Summary of Product Characteristics (SmPC) of a new product at launch, or considered medically important and where additional information is required, are followed up by sending additional questionnaires to the prescribing GP. PEM is dynamic in nature and the types and nature of events may evolve during the course of the study following publications of, for example, case reports or regulatory concerns. Individual case reports are assessed for causality according to DSRU procedure, using

PLEASE REMOVE THIS SECTION OF THE FORM SO THAT THE BOTTOM HALF BECOMES ANONYMOUS AND KEEP FOR FUTURE REFRENCE IN THE EVENT OF FOLLOW-UP

DRUG SAFETY RESEARCH UNIT
PRESCRIPTION EVENT MONITORING

MEDICAL - IN CONFIDENCE

DR.

WOULD YOU PLEASE COMPLETE THIS QUESTIONNAIRE FOR:

WHO WAS PRESCRIBED

ON

Saad A W Shakir, FRCP (Glas & Ed),FFPM,MRCGP.
Bursledon Hall,
Southampton SO31 1AA
Telephone: (023) 80408600
We collect EVENT data

An EVENT is any new diagnosis, any reason for referral to a consultant or admission to hospital, any unexpected deterioration (or improvement) in a concurrent illness, any suspected drug reaction, any alteration of clinical importance in laboratory values or any other complaint which was considered of sufficient importance to enter in the patient's notes. Example: A broken leg is an EVENT.

Please indicate if you suspect an EVENT to be an adverse reaction to a drug.

These studies are conducted in accordance with the results of authorative discussions and the International Ethical Guidelines for Biomedical Research Involving Human Subjects prepared by the Council for International Organizations of Medical Sciences (CIOMS) in collaboration with the World Health Organization (WHO), Geneva 1993. The method of study also complies with the Guidelines on the practice of Ethics Committees in Medical Research Involving Human Subjects, as issued by the Royal College of Physicians of London (August 1996)

Your identification code for this patient*

Ref:

PLEASE RETURN THIS HALF OF THE FORM   Ref:

Your identification code for this patient*	
Sex:	Age at start of treatment:
Indication for prescribing	

Was the drug effective?   Yes ☐ No ☐ Don't Know ☐

Has the drug been stopped? Yes ☐ No ☐ Don't Know ☐

If 'YES' reason for stopping

Drug start date ___ / ___ / ___   Dose ___ mg/day

Date of last prescription ___ / ___ / ___

Drug stop date ___ / ___ / ___

Event Date	Dose mg/day	Events while taking this drug If none, please tick box ☐	Event Date	Events after stopping this drug If none, please tick box ☐

IF YOUR PATIENT HAS DIED: Date of death ___ / ___ / ___

Certified cause of death 1a ___

Underlying cause ___

	Yes	No	Don't know
1. Prior to taking celecoxib was there any history of dyspeptic symptoms or other upper gastrointestinal conditions?	☐	☐	☐
2. Were any NSAIDs prescribed in the 3 months prior to celecoxib?	☐	☐	☐
3. Were any of the following drugs prescribed during treatment with celecoxib?	☐	☐	☐

	Yes	No	Don't Know		Yes	No	Don't know
NSAIDs	☐	☐	☐	H2 antagonists/Proton pump inhibitors	☐	☐	☐
Misoprostol	☐	☐	☐	Antacids	☐	☐	☐
Aspirin	☐	☐	☐	Anticoagulants/Antiplatelet agents	☐	☐	☐

IMPORTANT: PLEASE INDICATE ANY EVENTS REPORTED TO CSM OR MANUFACTURER
This enables YOU to identify the patient in any future correspondence concerning this report

FIGURE 9.4 An example of a PEM Green Form questionnaire

four basic considerations (temporality, pharmacological plausibility, clinical and pathological characteristics of the event, exclusion of other possible causes) and classified according to one of five categories (probable, possible, unlikely, awaiting further information or not assessable).[27] All deaths reported as events for which a cause was not specified are followed up to try to establish the cause of death.

Confidentiality

All records and computer data are stored at the DSRU to maximise patient confidentiality, by irreversible anonymisation of patient identifiable data supplied by the PPD after the Green Form questionnaires have been sent, and the use of unique identifier codes supplied to the DSRU by the GP for any subsequent correspondence.[28]

Strengths and weaknesses of PEM

PEM monitors the safety of newly licensed medicines on a national scale and uses a non-interventional cohort design that does not interfere in the prescribing decisions of the practitioners, or specify strict inclusion criteria that occur within RCTs.[25] Thus, PEM provides information on a large cohort of patients representing actual general practice use of a study drug regardless of age, past medical history or concomitant medication. The main objective of PEM is to detect and quantify comparatively large risks that may go undetected in clinical trials, as mentioned previously. PEM prompts NHS primary care GP prescribers in England of the study drug during the data collection period to report all significant health related 'events' that have been recorded in each patient's notes following the initial prescription. By removing the need for GPs to give an opinion about the probability that any particular event might have been caused by the drug, PEM may identify reactions which neither the patient nor prescriber had suspected as being due to the drug being monitored, thus generating hypotheses regarding drug alerts or 'signals' that may be of public health interest.[29,30]

PEM is the only method of postmarketing surveillance that has been shown to be capable of evaluating the safety of new drugs in cohorts that are frequently over 10 000 patients. PEM exploits the unique nature of the NHS in that nearly all patients are allocated a GP, who has access to primary and secondary care medical records. Unlike spontaneous reporting schemes, PEM enables examination of the time relationship between exposure and events because information is collected on both the number of events (numerator) and the duration of exposure for each patient (denominator). Thus, PEM provides estimates of incidence measures of multiple outcomes (events) associated with drug use.

Achieving high response rates is an important issue in any postmarketing surveillance study and the average response rate for 93 PEM studies to date is 55.6%. Selection bias may be introduced by falling GP response rates to postal surveys,[31] and as in any observational study dependent on third party reporting, outcome misclassification is possible. Under-reporting of events, including serious or fatal events, is also possible in PEM. PEM does not include hospital prescriptions, and it is not possible to estimate prescription adherence that may lead to an underestimate of the measure of effect, or to a false conclusion regarding any possible associations between the drug and any outcomes. Prescribers may be influenced by ADRs reported in the literature, especially for drugs launched first elsewhere. For PEM, such publicity bias is minimised because the prescriber is requested to report *all* events and not to determine causation. As GPs are more likely to recognise and report adverse events in the first months of treatment there may also be a reporting bias. This may have the effect of skewing the distribution of events, so that relative excess is apparent during early months of treatment. Nevertheless, this is likely to be observed in all PEM studies.

Signal detection in PEM

The identification of drug safety alerts or 'signals' is a complex process in which the identification of previously unknown associations between a suspected drug and an ADR, causality and quantification are closely related. In any postmarketing surveillance system, routine clinical appraisal of event reports facilitates the earliest possible generation of hypotheses regarding drug safety signals.

Quantitative methods

PEM uses several computerised 'automated' approaches to generating signals, including calculation and ranking of rates – also called incidence densities (IDs) – and ID differences between the first (ID_1) and subsequent months of treatment or observation, e.g. months 2 to 6 (ID_2). The ID difference (ID_1-ID_2), together with the 99% confidence interval (CI) is calculated in order to test the null hypothesis that the rate for the event is not changing over time. Where the difference (and 99% CI) excludes zero, this may signal the possibility that the event is associated with the drug.[32] This is important for adverse events, since most drug reactions occur shortly after starting therapy. Although use of the 99% CI means that initially more potential drug safety signals are identified as significant, this enables the capture of more signals (although one is less certain about the true estimate of risk). Stratification of IDs according to age, sex, indication, pattern of use or from additional questions regarding important risk factors also enables calculation of ratios of IDs (plus standard 95% CI) for selected periods (most relevant to the drug under study) which can be used to generate hypotheses of safety signals in subgroups of the study population. Other quantitative methods of signal generation in PEM include looking at the most common reasons for stopping, comparisons of 'Reasons for withdrawal' and IDs.

Qualitative clinical methods

In PEM, each Green Form undergoes initial evaluation by research fellows to screen for adverse events that may possibly be related to drug exposure. The types of events to be screened may be (but not always) directed from published literature, or by specific request from external sources such as the regulatory authority or manufacturer. These will include the following.

- Medically important adverse events:
  - reported during pre-marketing development
  - reported during postmarketing in other countries (for products launched elsewhere before the UK)
  - for the therapeutic class (*if appropriate*)
  - considered to be possibly associated with the product during the PEM study.
- Reports of overdose and suicide.
- Any other adverse events deemed to be of medical importance by the DSRU during the PEM study.
- Any events included on the list of rare and iatrogenic adverse drug reactions (RAIDR) compiled by the DSRU. These are rare adverse events which are serious and a high proportion is due to drugs, for example agranulocytosis, anaphylaxis and Stevens-Johnson Syndrome.

This qualitative assessment takes into consideration a number of points, including temporality, dechallenge/rechallenge and biological plausibility (among others).[27] Although automated detection methods help to speed up the process of identifying signals, these methods should only be regarded as tools to supplement careful clinical evaluation.

Developments in signal detection

Postmarketing pharmacovigilance systems often use different

mathematical tools to identify signals. The underlying principle is to examine the disproportionality in the reporting of events observed for a drug compared to that expected in the background (according to other drugs within the database).[33]

Statistical methods used in the quantitative analysis of anecdotal spontaneous ADRs at the MHRA (and other regulatory or manufacturers' databases) include the use of proportional reporting ratios (PRRs).[34] This technique tests the null hypothesis that the proportion of individual adverse reactions reported for a drug of interest compared to the rest of the database does not change, with a predefined statistical criterion representing a signal. The PEM and MHRA systems both use hierarchical dictionaries that enable reports to be coded onto their respective databases. The use of an automated system to complement the process of identification of possible safety signals in PEM has also been developed in recent years.[30] In addition to PRRs, ID rate ratios (IRR) are being utilised as a tool for signal detection in PEM to highlight those events with a rate that is unexpectedly different from the background event rate calculated for other drugs in the database.[35] These IRRs may be calculated for the whole PEM database, or for subgroups of patients according to certain characteristics (e.g. age or sex), if appropriate.

The strengths and limitations of such signal detection methods have been discussed in detail elsewhere,[33,34] but consideration should be given to choice of drugs to be used when making the comparison, the dictionary level, the time periods within which to compare, and that events may be indication-related or associated with the underlying disease. It is important to remember that whilst these quantitative approaches appear to yield objective estimates of risk and allude to hypotheses of safety signals, the detection of signals within a database cannot be taken as conclusive evidence for clinical differences in the safety profiles of drugs within any therapeutic class of medicine. Signal detection must not detract from, or be viewed as a substitute for, individual case analysis; further details of individual cases are necessary to confirm or refute that a possible safety signal exists, as well as obtain useful information on possible risk factors.

Signal detection is still in its infancy but has the potential to offer elegant statistical approaches to complement signal generation in pharmacovigilance. Worldwide, a number of different algorithms for selecting signals are being utilised or are under development. The World Health Organization (WHO) Uppsala Monitoring Centre

(UMC) in Sweden uses a number of different strategies using the Bayesian Confidence Propagation Neural Network (BCPNN) to manage the data in the WHO Drug Monitoring Database.[36,37] In the UK, the MHRA is developing a scoring system to aid signal prioritisation for spontaneous ADR data[38] as well as assessing the application of other data-mining algorithms.[39]

Dissemination of DSRU findings

Peer review publications

There are 93 PEM studies on the database, with a median cohort size of 10935 patients. Reports are sent to the UK regulatory body MHRA, the EMEA's Committee for Proprietary Medicinal Products (CPMP) Pharmacovigilance Working Party and the manufacturer whose product has been under surveillance during the PEM study monitoring period.

The DSRU aims to publish the results of all studies undertaken in peer reviewed journals, outlining items of specific interest identified during the analysis. These published papers are circulated to all pharmacovigilance centres, academics and professionals involved in drug safety activities. Feedback to GPs is achieved through a biannual DSRU Newsletter and lay interpretation of study results are displayed on the Patient Focus section of the website (http://www.dsru.org) together with the list of publications. The DSRU also presents abstracts of selected studies at national and international conferences.

Education and training

In addition to publishing in the medical and scientific literature, part of the DSRU's remit is to educate and disseminate information at national and international scientific meetings. Training courses and symposia are provided annually, including courses designed for the Drug Safety Module which forms part of the Faculty of Pharmaceutical Medicine's Higher Medical Training programme for pharmaceutical physicians. Participants in the training courses include personnel from the pharmaceutical industry, regulators, academics and other healthcare professionals. As a service to GPs two educational distance learning modules on the safety of medicines at Introductory and Advanced level are available free on the DSRU website. These modules were developed to increase awareness and understanding of ADRs as an important and potentially preventable cause of disease and to promote understanding of and effective use of safety monitoring schemes. These modules have been extended to pharmacists, with further extensions planned for nurses.

Conclusion

The Yellow Card spontaneous reporting system and PEM provide complementary information on hazards associated with medicines. There are important differences in the type of data collected in PEM compared with the Yellow Card Scheme, the most important being that the majority of events reported in PEM will **not** be adverse reactions and should **not** be treated as spontaneous adverse reaction reports. Nevertheless, both postmarketing systems are able to generate hypotheses regarding safety signals. PEM provides estimates of common to rare events whilst the Yellow Card reporting scheme is able to detect signals of very rare events because of the size of the population being monitored. With an increasing number of completed studies, PEM provides opportunities for hypothesis testing and comparative studies.

The underlying principle in both systems is based on the assessment and management of risk: a continuous cycle of identifying, analysing, prioritising, resolving and monitoring risk according to all the available levels of evidence (spontaneous case reports, case series, observational studies and randomised controlled trials). Whatever the source of evidence, one cannot escape the basic requirement that the event must be recorded and reported, and the Yellow Card Scheme and PEM provide a means to do just that. Education and training of reporters is encouraged and provided by both the MHRA and the DSRU, although greater emphasis is also required at the undergraduate level.[40]

The importance of reporting adverse events is reflected in the growing number of new international guidelines, which plan to incorporate pharmacovigilance and risk management throughout the life-cycle plan of a product (pre- *and* postmarketing) as well as standardisation of international adverse event reporting. Legislation has paved the way for the rapid transmission of data between European Union regulatory authorities and for the standardisation of adverse event reporting. The EUDRA Vigilance System is the next big step in the process of pharmacovigilance for licensed medicinal products in Europe.[41] Revision of existing and development of additional guidelines at the EU level (Volume 9 A of the Rules governing Medicinal Products, 25 January 2007), also set out clearer steps for the expectations of the conduct of pharmacovigilance by pharmaceutical companies.

References

1. Pocock SJ. Size of cancer clinical trials and stopping rules. *Br J Cancer* 1978; **38**: 757–66.
2. Pocock SJ. Current issues in the design and interpretation of clinical trials. *Br Med J (Clin Res Ed)* 1985; **290**: 39–42.
3. Raine J, Davis S. Spontaneous Reporting – UK. In: Mann RD, Andrews EB, editors. *Pharmacovigilance*. Chichester, UK: John Wiley & Sons Ltd; 2002: 195–208.
4. Lee A, Bateman DN, Edwards C, Smith JM, Rawlins MD. Reporting of adverse drug reactions by hospital pharmacists: pilot scheme. *BMJ* 1997; **315**: 519.
5. Davis S, Coulson R. Community pharmacists reporting of suspected ADRs: (1) The first year of the yellow card demonstration scheme. *Pharmaceutical J* 1999; **263**: 786–8.
6. Morrison-Griffiths S, Pirmohamed M. Specialist nurse reporting of adverse drug reactions. *Professional Nurse* 2000; **15**: 300–304.
7. MHRA. Report of an Independent Review of Access to the Yellow Card Scheme. http://www.mhra.gov.uk/home/groups/comms-ic/documents/websiteresources/con2015008.pdf (accessed 14 March 2006). www.mhra.gov.uk 2004. London, The Stationery Office.
8. Brown EG. Dictionaries and Coding in Pharmacovigilance. In: Talbot J, Waller PC, editors. *Stephens' Detection of New Adverse Drug Reactions*. Chichester, UK: John Wiley & Sons Ltd; 2004. pp. 533–57.
9. Hazel L, Shakir SAW. Under-reporting of adverse drug reactions: a systematic review. *Drug Saf* 2006; **29**: 385–96.
10. Smith CC, Bennett PM, Pearce HM, Harrison PI, Reynolds DJ, Aronson JK, Grahame-Smith DG. Adverse drug reactions in a hospital general medical unit meriting notification to the Committee on Safety of Medicines. *Br J Clin Pharmacol* 1996; **42**: 423–9.
11. Heeley E, Riley J, Layton D, Wilton LV, Shakir SA. Prescription-Event monitoring and reporting of adverse drug reactions. *Lancet* 2001; **358**: 1872–3.
12. Deehan A, Templeton L, Taylor C, Drummond C, Strang J. The effect of cash and other financial inducements on the response rate of general practitioners in a national postal study. *Br J Gen Pract* 1997; **47**: 87–90.
13. Waller P, Lee E. Responding to Drug Safety issues. *Pharmacoepidemiol Drug Saf* 1999; **8**: 535–52.
14. National Audit Office. *Safety, Quality, Efficacy: Regulating medicines in the*

UK (Full Report). http://www.nao.gov.uk/publications/nao_reports/02-03/0203255.pdf. HC 255 2002–2003. 16-1-2003. London, The Stationery Office.

15. Great Britain Parliament House of Commons Committee of Public Accounts. Safety, quality, efficacy regulating medicines in the UK twenty-sixth report of session 2002–03. 505. 26-6-2003. London, The Stationery Office.

16. Egberts TC, Smulders M, de Koning FH, Meyboom RH, Leufkens HG. Can adverse drug reactions be detected earlier? A comparison of reports by patients and professionals. *BMJ* 1996; **313**: 530–1.

17. van Grootheest K, de Graaf L, de Jong-van den Berg LT. Consumer adverse drug reaction reporting: a new step in pharmacovigilance? *Drug Saf* 2003; **26**: 211–17.

18. Boseley S. Patients get the right to report drug side-effects. *The Guardian.* Wednesday 5 May 2004.

19. Medawar C, Herxheimer A, Bell A, Jofre S. Paroxetine, *Panorama* and user reporting of ADRs: consumer intelligence matters in clinical practice and postmarketing surveillance. *Int J Risk and Safety in Medicine* 2002; **15**: 161–9.

20. National Co-ordinating Centre for Research Methodology. RM05/JH30 – Evaluation of patient reporting to the yellow card system. http://pcpoh.bham.ac.uk/publichealth/nccrm/invitations.htm (accessed 18 May 2006). Department of Public Health and Epidemiology; 2006.

21. Casiday R, Cresswell T, Wilson D, Panter-Brick C. A survey of UK parental attitudes to the MMR vaccine and trust in medical authority. *Vaccine* 2006; **24**: 177–84.

22. Legemaate J. The CIOMS guidelines for biomedical research involving human subjects. *Eur J Health Law* 1994; **1**: 161–5.

23. Royal College of Physicians of London. Guidelines on the practice of Ethical Committees in Medical Research involving Human Subjects. 1996.

24. GMC. Frequently asked questions supplement to: Confidentiality: Protecting and Providing Information. Page 9. 2004. General Medical Council, 178 Great Portland Street, London, W1W 5JE. gmc-uk.org.

25. Shakir S. Prescription-Event Monitoring. In: Strom BL, editor. *Pharmacoepidemiology.* Chichester, UK: John Wiley & Sons Ltd; 2005. pp. 203–16.

26. Strom B. Sample size considerations for pharmacoepidemiology studies. In: Strom B, editor. *Pharmacoepidemiology.* Chichester, UK: John Wiley & Sons; 1994.

27. Shakir SAW. Causality and Correlation in Pharmacovigilance. In: Talbot J, Waller PC, editors. *Stephens' Detection of New Adverse Drug Reactions.* Chichester, UK: John Wiley & Sons Ltd; 2004. pp. 329–43.

28. Multi-Centre Research Ethics Committees Guidance Notes. Examples of enquiries and surveys in the public interest where no reference to a Research Ethics Committee is necessary. http://www.corec.org.uk/wordDocs/Guidenotes.doc. Appendix C, p. 21 (accessed 19 October 2000).

29. Wilton LV, Stephens MD, Mann RD. Visual field defects associated with vigabatrin: observational cohort study. *BMJ* 1999; **319**: 1165–6.

30. Heeley E, Wilton LV, Shakir SA. Automated signal generation in prescription-event monitoring. *Drug Saf* 2002; **25**: 423–32.
31. Key C, Layton D, Shakir SA. Results of a postal survey of the reasons for non-response by doctors in a Prescription-Event Monitoring study of drug safety. *Pharmacoepidemiol Drug Saf* 2002; **11**: 143–8.
32. Stephens MD. The diagnosis of adverse medical events associated with drug treatment. *Adverse Drug React Acute Poisoning Rev* 1987; **6**: 1–35.
33. Meyboom RH, Egberts AC, Edwards IR, Hekster YA, de Koning FH, Gribnau FW. Principles of signal detection in pharmacovigilance. *Drug Saf* 1997; **16**: 355–65.
34. Hauben M, Zhou X. Quantitative methods in pharmacovigilance: focus on signal detection. *Drug Saf* 2003; **26**: 159–86.
35. Layton D, Heeley E, Shakir SA. Identification and evaluation of a possible signal of exacerbation of colitis during rofecoxib treatment, using Prescription-Event Monitoring data. *J Clin Pharm Ther* 2004; **29**: 171–81.
36. Lindquist M, Stahl M, Bate A, Edwards IR, Meyboom RH. A retrospective evaluation of a data mining approach to aid finding new adverse drug reaction signals in the WHO international database. *Drug Saf* 2000; **23**: 533–42.
37. Stahl M, Lindquist M, Edwards IR, Brown EG. Introducing triage logic as a new strategy for the detection of signals in the WHO Drug Monitoring Database. *Pharmacoepidemiol Drug Saf* 2004; **13**: 355–63.
38. Heeley E, Waller P, Moseley J. Testing and implementing signal impact analysis in a regulatory setting: results of a pilot study. *Drug Saf* 2005; **28**: 901–06.
39. Roux E, Thiessard F, Fourrier A, Begaud B, Tubert-Bitter P. Evaluation of statistical association measures for the automatic signal generation in pharmacovigilance. *IEEE Trans Inf Technol Biomed* 2005; **9**: 518–27.
40. Cox AR, Marriott JF, Wilson KA, Ferner RE. Adverse drug reaction teaching in UK undergraduate medical and pharmacy programmes. *J Clin Pharm Ther* 2004; **29**: 31–35.
41. European Commission and the EMEA. EudraVigilance. pharmacovigilance in the EU. http://eudravigilance.emea.eu.int (accessed 23 March 2004).

10 The future: service changes and challenges for data linkage

CHRISTINE BOND AND CHRISTINE CLARKE

This chapter provides an overview of recent, current and imminent service changes. It builds on some of the topics introduced in earlier chapters, considers their impact on the generation of comprehensive routine datasets and highlights some of the challenges surrounding these.

Introduction

Information technology is integral to many services that the general public use every day. For example banking, booking a holiday, or paying one's tax bill are all managed using various new technologies based on cards embedded with chips, digital strips, or Internet or intranet communications. In this regard the use of technology in health has not kept up with other industries, particularly those in the private sector. An ever-increasing number of systems and databases have developed, but in an opportunistic rather than a planned way and until recently there has been little opportunity to link these different databases for the direct and indirect benefit of patient care. This chapter considers some of these datasets, used at individual practitioner level, and reflects on the potential value of linking these datasets, and some of the challenges this might bring.

Datasets as part of routine practice in primary care
General practice

In primary care the main datasets which are in use are hosted at either the individual GP or community pharmacy level. Both of the professions have to some extent both benefited and suffered from the development of systems in a commercial environment, which has resulted in continual research and upgrading of systems to remain competitive, but also in many different systems (e.g. VISION, EMIS), with different functionality and the obvious drawbacks associated with this.

The exception to this scenario is in general practice in Scotland where there was a central decision taken in 1984 to invest in a software system known as GPASS (General Practice Administration System Scotland) which was made available to all GPs as part of an attractive financial package. As a result approximately 80% of all GPs currently use the GPASS system, which has continued to be revised and developed in line with the commercially available packages. The advantage of this is that it is possible to collate at a national level prescribing data for the majority of patients in Scotland, rather than dispensing data (which is the basis for PACT, SPA and PRISMs data; *see* Chapter 7). A dedicated unit, based at the University of Aberdeen, originally the GPASS Data Evaluation Project, and now known as Primary Care Clinical Informatics Research Unit (PCCIU-R), collects data electronically at six monthly intervals from all practices. The data is used for individualised practice feedback, particularly for the management of chronic diseases.

As often is the case, the incentive for practices to use the new system was to facilitate their current practice. Therefore the original data collected at GP level was based on information required for administration purposes, such as repeat prescribing, or booking appointments. Recently it has evolved to have more clinical functions, and includes all acute and repeat prescribing, morbidity and provides decision support. The comprehensiveness of the data, and therefore its value as both a robust national dataset and potential use in research, has been questioned. To counter this a subset of practices, originally known as CMR practices (continuous morbidity recording), were recruited who agreed to record data comprehensively on patient demography, prescribing, morbidity, physiological measurements and health promotion activity. This provided a useful cross-sectional description of national activity for research and monitoring purposes, known as Practice Team Information (personal communication Dr Colin Simpson, PCCIU-R).

Community pharmacy

Patient Medication Records (PMRs) first emerged in community pharmacy in the 1990s as part of a negotiated contracted process which was the first initial step to move community pharmacy from a technical dispensing paradigm to a more clinically delivered service. Initially pharmacists were required to maintain records on a minimum of 50 patients in order to meet the required PMR criterion to activate payment of the 'Professional Allowance'. (Overall a package of different criteria had to be met; these also included the display of health promotion leaflets, production of a practice leaflet and in Scotland participation in Clinical Audit.)

Initially a paper, card-based, system was the norm but quickly commercial software systems became available linking the labelling function of pharmacy computer systems to the patient record and pharmacies quickly built up large datasets of patients, including valuable patient histories of medication dispensed and collected (as opposed to prescribed). As up to 20% of prescriptions are variously claimed not to be dispensed, these records of dispensed medication at an individual patient level were unique, but failed to deliver their full potential as they were not linked to GP held patient records. Although 80–90% of patients are known to use the same pharmacy for all their medication, the public are free to get a prescription dispensed from any pharmacy with an NHS contract and so as pharmacies were not networked (other than within some multiple groups), there was a further lost opportunity for a meaningful and comprehensive dataset.

Developments in primary care

Most recently policy documents in the UK have encouraged developments pursuing the mantra of increased patient convenience and improved access to medicines. One aspect of this is that across all the home countries plans for the electronic transmission of prescriptions (ETP), from GP to pharmacy, are being progressed thus removing the inconvenient need for the patient to physically obtain a paper prescription from the GP, perhaps when there was no other reason to visit the surgery premises. ETP pilots have been conducted and evaluated in England; problems of electronic communication across a multiplicity of software providers in both pharmacy and GP settings have been identified and overcome. Within the new community pharmacy contracts (introduced in England from 2005, in Scotland from 2006) ETP is a future integral component and is paving the way for what has become known as repeat dispensing from community pharmacists.

Further linking of the technical repeat dispensing service to a clinical function, known as the Chronic Medicine Service (CMS Scotland) or Medicine Use Review (MUR England) is envisaged. However, for this to be of maximum benefit pharmacists will need to have electronic access to the patient's medical record (held in the GP surgery) both at a read and write level. Even at the most basic level, the ability of the GP to quickly determine if this patient has been collecting their prescribed medicine at the appropriate intervals would greatly inform ongoing clinical assessment and management.

At the time of writing, community pharmacists across the UK are being connected to the NHS net with anticipation of the benefits this will bring. In Scotland this is now complete and is ongoing in England as part of the Connecting for Health initiative.

The secondary care setting

Electronic prescribing is now well established in many hospitals in the United Kingdom.

In some hospitals electronic prescribing developed as an off-shoot of the pharmacy stock-control/dispensing record system and in others it developed as a module in a hospital-wide IT system that saw prescribing of drugs as essentially similar to other order processes such as the ordering of laboratory tests or X-rays. In some institutions, so-called vertical systems have been developed that deal with the needs of one specific group of patients; for example, cancer patients or patients in intensive care. Such systems are usually stand-alone systems. In the long term, hospitals need integrated information management systems that allow users to access all relevant information for a single patient. Moreover, such a system will need to be able to link to a centrally held electronic care record that could, for example, contain details of treatment that the patient has received in other hospitals. This is the vision that is currently being pursued by Connecting for Health, the Department of Health agency that is responsible for implementation of the National Programme for IT in England. Over the next 10 years, it is scheduled to connect over 30 000 GPs in England to almost 300 hospitals and give patients access to their personal health and care information, transforming the way the NHS works.

Dictionary of Medicines and Devices (dm+d)

The development and implementation of a standard dictionary for drugs and devices was a major step forward because it meant that it was possible to pass information from one system to another. In simple terms, the dm+d provides a unique code for each medicine and device along with a textual description of the item. It covers medicines and devices used in both acute and primary care and it is integrated with another terminology – SNOMED clinical terms – that provides unique codes for clinical terms and concepts. When prescribing and hospital pharmacy stock control systems were first developed they relied on a variety of different coding systems for drugs. These were usually different from the coding schemes used in community pharmacies and different again from those in GP prescribing systems. As they were stand-alone systems this was not a problem but when, for example, something as apparently simple as the integration of a prescribing system with a pharmacy system was contemplated it became essential for the two systems to use the same coding systems for medicines. For this reason considerable resources were invested in the development of the dm+d.[1,2]

Computerised pharmacy stock control systems of yesteryear allowed identification of which products had been issued to which wards. This was useful for product recalls and for simple analyses of prescribing trends. However, pharmacy IT systems that are an integral part of the hospital IT systems can offer much more. In the first place, there are considerable benefits for day-to-day running of the pharmacy; for example, patient details can be drawn directly from the patient administration system (PAS) instead of being rekeyed by pharmacy staff. This saves time and avoids the risks of transcription errors. Clinical pharmacists can also check laboratory tests online before issuing or prescribing a drug. Recent developments, such as the picture archiving and communication system (PACS) mean that clinical images (X-rays, scans, photographs) are also available to authorised users.

In some places, e.g. the Hope Hospital, Salford, this has been taken one step further – not only is the whole hospital served by an integrated IT system, but also GPs in the locality.[3] The benefits of this type of linkage are considerable. For example, there is the practical benefit of not having to rewrite patient details repeatedly and also the ability to send discharge summaries, including medication summaries, to GPs without delay. Such systems also have the facility for GPs to refer patients to hospital specialists. In addition, laboratory test results, including diagnostic imaging, are available to all appropriate parties at all times. Access is controlled by password; for example, a ward clerk has access to demographic data but not clinical data. In this respect it could be argued that this type of system is more secure than the previous paper-based systems.

NHS care records service

In a further development the information held in the hospital IT system will be ultimately linked to records held in a national database of NHS care records. The way in which this will work is that a summary of the patient's care and clinical history will be held on a national database known as the 'spine' to ensure that particularly important patient information is always accessible. This will include data such as name, address, NHS number and date of birth, and clinical information such as allergies, adverse reactions to drugs and details of any visits to A&E. Detailed records including medical conditions, medication, operations, tests, X-rays, scans and other results will be held locally and links to local information will be available from the summary record. Thus, each NHS care record will be formed from information held in a number of places, which is automatically brought together when it is needed.[4]

Clearly, this system will amass vast amounts of electronic data and this will open up new possibilities and pose new challenges. We are already beginning to see some of the types of information that can be extracted from these systems, but, in future, sophisticated data-warehousing and data-mining tools will create many new possibilities.

Potential applications of electronic datasets

Well-developed hospital IT systems of today allow prescribing data to be interrogated to distinguish previously unrecognised patterns of drug usage and to identify at-risk patients. One example of this is a study of people taking long-term corticosteroids.[5] It is generally accepted that people receiving long-term corticosteroid treatment should also receive prophylactic treatment for osteoporosis. In this study, the prescribing data set was used to identify all patients receiving long-term corticosteroid treatment. From this subset it was possible to identify electronically those who were/were not receiving prophylactic treatment for osteoporosis. Such measures can be applied over time to monitor adherence to local policy and to identify areas where remedial action is required.

More sophisticated analyses are possible if the prescribing dataset can be linked to others, such as the pathology dataset. An example of this is a study that linked statin prescriptions to total cholesterol measurement.[6] In this way the effectiveness of statin treatment in a large population sample can be measured. This study showed that 75% of people had a satisfactory response to statin treatment and the remaining 25% could be identified. It also identified a group of people with elevated cholesterol who were not receiving statin treatment.

In the USA similar dedicated exercises have shown the value of linking datasets. For example, Bond and Raehl have linked the National Clinical Pharmacy Database (data from 1109 hospitals) and the Medicare hospital database (717 396 Medicare patients in 955 hospitals). They argue that studies of this type (very large numbers) are not subject to the biases of patient populations, physical facilities, structure and process or intervener's bias – as might occur in individual sites. They have, for example, been able to show that in hospitals without pharmacy-managed heparin management, death rates were 11.41% higher, and length of stay was 10% higher.[7] Results were similar for warfarin.[7]

These examples show that prescribing data can be linked with other datasets. It is easy to see how many more record-linkage initiatives could be useful, e.g. prescribing data could be linked with diagnostic codes or with other interventions. The advantage of doing it this way, is that, instead of trawling through medical records, large amounts of data can be searched and linked so that valid inferences can be drawn. In turn, this kind of information could inform operational decisions and strategic policy-making.

Future challenges to data capture and linkage
Nurse prescribing
Again with the declared primary purpose of improving access to medicines for the benefit of patients, there have been incremental

moves across the UK to increase the types of professionals authorised to write NHS prescriptions (see also earlier chapters). Initially, and following the Crown Report on nurse prescribing,[8] this development was based on providing a formal mechanism for nurses to prescribe a restricted range of products such as dressings and basic medicines including simple laxatives and analgesics, the choice of which had been effectively their clinical responsibility for many years, but for which they had needed to get a doctor's authorising signature. Nurse prescribing on a pilot basis was introduced in 1994.

Building on this, extended nurse prescribing was introduced in 2001, and under this regulation suitably trained nurses were allowed to provide a wider range of drugs and dressings including some medicines previously only available on a doctor's prescription. The clinical areas targeted were: minor ailments, minor injuries, health promotion and palliative care.

Further regulatory changes have extended the nurse practitioners' formulary to include an even wider range of drugs and specific indications, previously the sole domain of the medical profession. It is anticipated that the most recent changes[9] will make virtually the whole *BNF* available to specifically trained nurses, to prescribe within their own professional competence.

However, no systematic study has been conducted of the method of recording nurse prescribing and the comprehensiveness of individual medical records in this regard.

Nurses have also had their prescribing rights extended by other regulatory changes such as supplementary prescribing and Patient Group Directions which are described separately below.

The Crown Report: PGDs and supplementary prescribing

In the late 1990s, Dr June Crown was asked again to chair a group whose final recommendations would have major implications on the supply and administration of medicines. The rationale for convening the group was that once again it was perceived that practice was developing ahead of the regulatory framework. In particular nurses in the secondary care setting were acting autonomously in decision making with regards to the supply and administration of medicine. As a result of Part 1 of the second Crown Report[10] Patient Group Directions were introduced in 1999[11] to provide a more robust legal framework for the supply and administration of drugs by nurses, in both primary and secondary care, in situations where direct personal involvement of a medical practitioner may not be required for a 'prescription only' medicine. Examples of such drugs include vaccines, or dressings, or potentially antiviral treatments for use in an influenza pandemic. Increasingly other professionals, including pharmacy and chiropody, have also become involved. For example, pharmacists can supply smoking cessation products on the NHS to patients normally not allowed to purchase the products under the OTC licence. Part of the PGD regulation requires an audit trail to be maintained via appropriate record keeping, but the specification of a mechanism whereby this record would be linked to other records about the patient is up to local organisations. As a result, and probably more in primary care, medically held records are increasingly incomplete.

The second part of the Crown Report resulted in the introduction of more far reaching changes.[12] The supplementary prescribing regulation was passed by the UK Government in 2003;[13] this amendment to the Medicines Act allows pharmacists and nurses to undertake the long term prescribing of drugs for a patient following an initial medical diagnosis. Most of the drugs in the *BNF* are allowed to be prescribed within the framework of a Clinical Management Plan (CMP). The CMP has to be agreed jointly between the pharmacist, nurse, patient and responsible medical doctor and it specifies exactly the authorisation being delegated to the supplementary prescriber, e.g. change of drug dose in accordance with clinical signs and symptoms, change of drugs within and across therapeutic class and sub-class. Once again adequate record keeping is mandatory, but there is no currently available information detailing the extent to which these records are currently linked into any central electronic record held on the patient. Most recently, other healthcare professionals such as physiotherapists and radiographers have also acquired supplementary prescribing rights, adding further challenges to maintaining a single comprehensive patient record.

Independent prescribing

Most recently independent prescribing rights were granted to both nurses and pharmacists in 2006. Training curricula and frameworks are currently being agreed and this regulation has yet to be fully implemented. However, it clearly creates further challenges to maintaining comprehensive records.

Direct supply projects

Finally, there is also the further permutation, commonly known as 'direct supply'. Unlike the previous innovations, which applied to all NHS settings, this only applies to primary care, and even more specifically to the community pharmacy. Direct supply is the process by which community pharmacists can prescribe on the NHS a range of products for so-called minor ailments to patients who would normally be exempt from prescription charges and for conditions which pharmacists are competent to diagnose and manage. This system developed because of the belief that many GP consultations were only to meet a need for a free supply of medicine on prescription, rather than needing the GP's medical expertise. In many ways direct supply projects are not unlike a PGD except there is less administrative development and approval, and the medicines involved are those which the pharmacist could normally legally sell.

POM to P to GSL

In most countries, the supply of medicines is controlled by their legal classification. In the UK there are three broad classes of medicines known as prescription only medicines (POM), pharmacy medicines (P) and General Sales List medicines (GSL). Initially prescription only medicines could only be supplied if prescribed by a doctor (with the exception of a short list of drugs available on dental prescription), pharmacy medicines which had to be either sold directly by or under the supervision of a pharmacist, and GSL medicines which could be supplied from any retail outlet. Thus, with the exception of the dentally prescribed products, the more potent medicines (classified as POM) were prescribed by a doctor and the patient's record, held either in the primary or secondary care, would be complete (within the caveats and limitations already described).

The moves to increase the options for the supply of POMs, involving other professions, have already been described above. However, other changes affecting record keeping and comprehensiveness of records have also been ongoing. Since 1984 the need to restrict so many medicines to prescription only control has been questioned. Extensive use of medicines within a POM environment has provided evidence of safety in use beyond the original clinical trial data. Pressure on national prescribing budgets and the wish of the pharmaceutical industry to extend the commercial life of products once their patent has expired has resulted in a move to gradually deregulate a wide range of products from POM initially to P, and often ultimately to GSL level. Since 1984, when the first products were deregulated (the non-steroidal anti-inflammatory drug ibuprofen, the anti-diarrhoeal loperamide and the topical steroid hydrocortisone) over 70 products/ drug entities have been 'switched'. These changes were originally focused on either new treatments to treat symptoms traditionally managed in the pharmacy setting, or were new indications for treatments already supplied through pharmacy. More recent changes have included 'new' treatment for 'new' conditions. An example of such a recent proposal is a consultation on the OTC availability of azithromycin for selected indications such as chlamydia.

POM	Prescribed by specified healthcare professional. Record kept.	Most professional control – least patient control hard to access.
P	Sold by or under supervision of pharmacist. Record rarely kept.	Sold by or under supervision of pharmacist. Record rarely kept.
GSL	Available from any sales outlet – includes petrol stations! Record not kept.	Easy to access most patient control – least professional control.

FIGURE 10.1 Changes in UK medicines classifications

Despite widespread concerns about safety there have been only a few problems in practice, resulting in drugs being re-regulated to a more restrictive classification. Detailed discussion of these is outside the scope of this text. However, the implications of the moves for record keeping are significant and relevant. To date no records are routinely kept of OTC product supplies. Within individual community pharmacies, some recording may be maintained for selected drugs, or selected patients, but within the GSL category there is no record keeping at all, and no professional input. The original three products deregulated in 1984 are now available from any shop, supermarket or garage, as are many more.

From the GP perspective the increasing range of potent drugs available for purchase may lead to several patient management problems if record keeping and record linkages are not addressed. It is known from limited research that GPs do not routinely ask about, and patients do not routinely provide, information on the non-prescribed products they are using. So for a hypothetical patient with either acute or chronic pain, a patient can both be prescribed analgesics and purchase them. Whilst some analgesic combinations may be safe and have increased overall pain control (e.g. paracetamol and an NSAID such as ibuprofen), other combinations, such as the taking of two different NSAIDs, might result in much greater incidence of well known and significant adverse events of NSAIDs. This is therapeutic duplication. Another problem is drug interactions; for example, the chronic pain patient who is buying OTC ibuprofen might also be taking antihypertensive medication; interaction between members of these therapeutic classes can be clinically significant and reduce the efficacy of the anti-hypertensive.

From the public health perspective there is a current increase in interest in pharmacovigilance studies (*see* Chapter 9). If there is not a recognised or universal system to record and monitor people who buy products OTC, including the potent newly deregulated medicines, it will be impossible to trace subjects in the event of a Drug Alert, or urgent drug safety message. Similarly the power to capture epidemiological data on large population of users, including evidence of side effects experienced, will be lost.

If a medicine has a P classification, the pharmacist has a professional responsibility for ensuring it is sold for use under appropriate circumstances in line with the OTC product licence. The RPSGB Code of Ethics provides detailed guidance on exactly how this should be done.[14] Ensuring safe and appropriate use means, for example, asking questions to check that the end user is not taking other drugs known to interact with the OTC products or result in therapeutic duplications (see earlier). It might also mean that it should only be used in the absence of contraindications such as age restrictions, co-morbidities, or patient states, e.g. pregnancy. Asking sufficient questions to confirm all of these, sometimes in the public context of the community pharmacy OTC setting, can be difficult and time consuming, and may be resisted by the patient who sees the acquisition of the product as a commercial exchange. Access to a full set of patient medical information, perhaps via a smart card or barcode, could obviate the need for such questioning and online decision support could alert the provider to any contraindicated supply such as is occurring under the present system. Small dedicated follow-up studies[15] have shown that, despite the pharmacist theoretically having responsibilities as outline above, in practice ibuprofen is being sold under contraindicated circumstances, being taken at too high a dose, and use is resulting in excess morbidity. Reasons for this are multifactorial and are currently being studied to see whether omissions are due to lack of knowledge, which is unlikely, or more associated with the dynamics of the pharmacist-customer interaction, or as is more often the case, the pharmacy assistant-customer interaction.

Notwithstanding the current shortcomings of the P classification, the problems are multiplied many more times once GSL status is conferred on a product. No routine information is collected on supplies of GSL medicines, even when made from a pharmacy, and when sales are made from a non-pharmacy outlet there is no opportunity for any healthcare professional input at the time of sale. Future ways of collecting this information may be possible as technology develops, but there is also the philosophical question as to whether or not this is appropriate, and possibly more consideration should be given to the GSL classification.

Out of hours services

A final service development to consider is the delivery of out of hours services in primary care. Until fairly recently all GPs had a responsibility to care for their patients 24 hours a day, seven days a week, throughout the year. Under this arrangement, there was no difference in the maintenance of a complete patient medical record whether treatment was in normal working hours or the middle of the night. In the 1990s, in response to a range of issues, out of hours services were generally centralised and delivered via private co-operatives of GPs. Subsequently this became formalised within the new GMS contract, and the responsibility for out of hours care is no longer that of the GP, but of the NHS. At local level, the GP co-operatives are now managed by the NHS. In practical terms, however, the centralisation of out of hours care, whether through co-operatives or the managed service, has resulted in the same challenge for the linkage of all care data to a central point. Ultimately a single electronic patient record will address this, but for the moment collation of a comprehensive dataset at individual patient level remains a challenge.

Some challenges

A single electronic patient record, linking all settings of care (tertiary, secondary, intermediate, primary, and the community) and all professionals remains the ideal solution. At the moment the home countries (England and Wales, and Scotland) are working incrementally towards this.[16, 17] However, although a case has been made for a system to link the records of new prescribers, OTC supplies and the GP held medical record, what might be the disadvantages of such a linkage?

In the first instance the linkage might appear technically challenging, but given the networking across most/all of the developed world in financial transactions, it is hard to believe that a technical solution would not be possible.

What would the main stakeholders think of such a proposal? Some evidence does exist to inform our thinking on a potential linkage between community pharmacists and general practice.[18] Pharmacists are generally very positive about the benefits of accessing the medical record of their patients to inform counselling on chronic disease, dispensing of prescriptions and provision of OTC advice. Ideally they would like access to the whole medical record, but they prioritise information on medication, allergies and diagnoses over physiological measurements and laboratory test results. They would be less enthusiastic about writing information on OTC purchases to a central record because of the workload involved, so this would need to be facilitated by automatic devices, e.g. a credit card swipe system.

GPs are more cautious about allowing pharmacists access to the whole medical records, being very aware of their responsibility to the patient and issues of confidentiality. However, removal of that unique responsibility during out of hours at their request has already set a precedent for the violability of this. An incremental approach with initial access to information such as the drug records would be a sensible way to build trust and confidence. Inevitably some GPs would not want to know about the OTC purchases, fearing that this would put the responsibility for OTC use onto them, so issues of accountability for the supply of these products would need to be clarified.

Patients likewise have some concerns about pharmacists, and more significantly pharmacy staff, accessing their records. However, again an incremental approach, perhaps initially with specific patient consent, could gradually build on and demonstrate the added value of the concept in terms of safe, cost effective and clinically effective use of drugs.

The above challenges cannot be ignored. Fears of the effect of scheduled and unscheduled down time on care, and the speed of data transfer, are all things still to be considered and balanced against each other.

Whilst the above findings are specific to the general practice-community pharmacy interface the principles would be transferable to the healthcare setting generally, and we need urgently but incrementally to move towards full electronic connectivity in the interests of better patient care.

The legislative and regulatory framework

Recognising the above technical and professional changes, as well as social changes which are outside the scope of this book, statutes have been passed in the UK to provide a robust legal framework within which professionals can operate.[19] The Data Protection Act 1998, the Human Rights Act 1998, the Freedom of Information Act 2000, and the Health and Social Care Act 2001 all have implications for the linkages of databases, although there is nothing in any of them which would prevent this as long as is it in the patient's interest.

The statutes do little more than formalise what has long been accepted as good clinical practice. For example, doctors have always had an incontrovertible right to access a patient's medical records, but on the understanding that this was purely in the interests of the patient. Breach of this confidentiality could result in legal action being taken, as well as disciplinary action by the professional regulators.

The question for other professionals as they increasingly take on clinical roles is whether or not they have a right to access patient's notes in the interests of the best clinical care of the patient, without seeking specific consent from the patient to do this. Research projects that have demonstrated the value of extended professional, non-medical, roles normally report seeking specific patient consent from the patient. Once these new roles become routine, and part of the NHS infrastructure, then there is no legal reason why patient consent should be sought.

Nonetheless, the law is not everything. Public opinion is important and we need to know to what extent patients will accept wider access to their notes and to be aware of any concerns they might have in order for these to be addressed.

Adequate encryption must be employed when transferring information across the web and patients must be reassured at the robustness of this. Given that most people already make purchases on the Internet, transmitting personal information such as credit card details, it is hard to see why, with careful explanation, that they could not be reassured about medical notes.

In the first instance it might be appropriate to respect patients' human rights and allow them to control this access, probably via the medical profession. As confidence and familiarity lead to acceptance of wider access to records we should aim for an ultimate scenario in which there is no longer any cumbersome requirement to seek this permission.

Conclusion

As healthcare provision evolves, professional boundaries blur and the generic healthcare worker emerges, it will become increasingly important for a single patient health record to be available to ensure appropriate treatment and use of prescribed and OTC drugs. Ideally the record should cross both professional and care setting interfaces so that there is two way communication across all stages of the patient journey. Patient education, reassurance and an incremental approach will be helpful in supporting the acceptance of this ideal. Technical solutions to overcome issues of workload and data security will be required, but will draw on experience in other areas such as finance. Ultimately linkage with social work and other community partners might be an option allowing proper team-work in the interests of better patient care.

References

1. Frosdick P and Dalton C. What is the dm+d and what will it mean for you and pharmacy practice? *Pharm J* 2004; **273**(7311): 199–200.
2. www.dmd.nhs.uk
3. Salford Royal Hospitals NHS Trust's Electronic Patient Record (EPR) Project. www.connectingforhealth.nhs.uk/casestudies/nhs/salfordrhnhst (accessed 16 January 2006).
4. NHS Care Records Service. www.connectingforhealth.nhs.uk/delivery/programmes/nhscrs (accessed 16 January 2006).

5. Collins NB, Beard RJ, Candlish CA, Worsley AJ. Osteoporosis assessment tool for Sunderland city hospitals. *Int J Pharmacy Practice* 2002; **10**(Suppl): R24.

6. Beard RJ, Candlish CA, Woulff L. 'Simvastatin in public health: A curious outcome?' (Poster presentation) 34th European Symposium on Clinical Pharmacy, Amsterdam, October 2005 Conference abstracts published in Pharmacy World and Science 2006/Clinical Pharmacy Europe in February.

7. Bond CA and Raehl CL. Pharmacist-provided anticoagulation management in United States hospitals: death rates, length of stay, Medicare charges, bleeding complications, and transfusions. *Pharmacotherapy* 2004; **8**: 953–63

8. Department of Health. *Report of the Advisory Group on Nurse Prescribing.* 1st Crown Report. London, HMSO; 1989.

9. Department of Health. Improving patients' access to medicines: A guide to implementing nurse and pharmacist independent prescribing within the NHS in England. London: HMSO; 2006.

10. Department of Health. *Review of the prescribing, supply and administration of medicines.* 2nd Crown Report Part 1. London: HMSO; 1999.

11. Statutory Instrument. No. 3189. The National Health Service (Charges for Drugs and Appliances) Amendment (No. 2) Regulations; 2000.

12. Department of Health. *Review of prescribing, supply and administration of medicines, final report.* London: HMSO; 1999.

13. Department of Health. Supplementary prescribing by nurses and pharmacists within the NHS in England, a guide for implementation. London: HMSO; 2003.

14. Royal Pharmaceutical Society of Great Britain. *Medicines, Ethics and Practice* Issue 30. London: RPSGB; 2006.

15. Sinclair, HK, Bond, CM, Hannaford, PC. Over the counter ibuprofen: how and why is it used? *IJPP* 2000; **8**: 121–7.

16. http://www.connectingforhealth.nhs.uk/ (accessed 28 November 2006).

17. NHS Scotland. Your emergency care summary; what does it mean for you? 2006.

18. Porteous T, Bond C, Robertson R, Hannaford P, Reiter E. Electronic transfer of prescription related information: comparing the views of patients, GPs and pharmacists. *Br J Gen Prac* 2003; **53**: 204–9.

19. Wingfield, J and Foster C. Consent and confidentiality. Legal implications of electronic transmission of prescriptions. *Pharmaceutical J* 2002; **269**: 328–31.

Index